*COST-CONTAINED
REGULATORY
COMPLIANCE*

COST-CONTAINED REGULATORY COMPLIANCE

For the Pharmaceutical, Biologics, and Medical Device Industries

SANDY WEINBERG

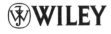

A JOHN WILEY & SONS, INC., PUBLICATION

For general information on our other products and services or for technical support, please contact our
Customer Care Department within the United States at (800) 762-2974, outside the United States at
(317) 572-3993 or fax (317) 572-4002.

Wiley also publishes its books in a variety of electronic formats. Some content that appears in print
may not be available in electronic formats. For more information about Wiley products, visit our web
site at www.wiley.com.

Library of Congress Cataloging-in-Publication Data:

Weinberg, Sandy, 1950–
    Cost-contained regulatory compliance : for the pharmaceutical, biologics, and medical device
industries / by Sandy Weinberg.
        p. ; cm.
    ISBN 978-0-470-55235-3 (cloth)
    1. Medical instruments and apparatus industry–United States–Cost control.   2. Medical instruments
and apparatus–Inspection–United States.   3. Pharmaceutical industry–United States–Cost
control.   4. Pharmaceutical industry–Inspection–United States.   5. United States. Food and Drug
Administration.   I. Title.
    [DNLM: 1. United States. Food and Drug Administration.   2. Drug Industry–economics–
United States.   3. Biotechnology–economics–United States.   4. Consumer Product Safety–
standards–United States.   5. Cost Control–methods–United States.   6. Equipment and Supplies–
economics–United States.   7. Quality Assurance, Health Care–economics–United States. QV 736]
    HD9994.U52W45 2011
    615.1068'1–dc22

                                                                                    2010028410

Printed in Singpore

oBook: 978-0-470-93351-0
ePDF: 978-0-470-93350-3
ePub: 978-1-118-00227-8

10 9 8 7 6 5 4 3 2 1

CONTENTS

PREFACE

In difficult economic times, the first rule of management is to conserve financial resources. In good economic times, the same rule prevails. Cost containment means less borrowing, greater flexibility, and higher profits.

But to the pharmaceutical, medical device, and biologics industries, cost containment has a significance that transcends financial considerations. The altruistic goal of these health-care industries is to bring therapeutics, preventatives, and quality-of-life enhancements to the public. In the United States and much of the world, the major impairment to that access is cost: Regardless of need, expensive drugs, vaccines, and devices are less available to the people who need them.

There are a number of expense centers that need careful monitoring and close cost control: manufacturing, distribution, research, and so forth. Somewhere on the list—perhaps not at the top of the potential amount of savings but high on the opportunity for control—is the cost of regulation. The investment necessary to maintain top-level quality assurance and control, and to demonstrate that level to outside government (or industry) reviewers are not without need, but often may be layered in fat appropriate for trimming. There may well be areas in which quality can be achieved and demonstrated at lower costs without losing credibility or control.

This book identifies eight proven strategies for containing the costs of regulatory compliance without sacrificing quality or safety. These are not techniques for fooling regulators, for shortcutting quality controls, or for risking public safety. Rather, these eight strategies address areas in which the pharmaceutical, biologics, and medical device industries have evolved approaches that add cost to the regulatory process without adding quality or safety. The strategies identify areas in which a lack of understanding or clarity of the letter and spirit of regulation has led to unnecessary and nonrequired industries standards that add nothing of value. Partially as a result of paranoia, partially because of FDA lack of clarity, and partially a result of evolutionary force ("most companies are testing 20 samples; let's test 25 just to be safe"; "they tested 25 at my old company; let's use 30 as a standard to avoid problems ..."), regulations seem to grow well beyond their original intent. While that growth seems harmless on the ground, it ultimately leads to reduced access for more and more patients—a cycle worth controlling.

The first part of this book defines the eight cost-containment strategies. An introductory chapter (Chapter 1) provides the theoretical framework and introduces the eight strategies.

Chapter 2 describes a very successful strategy based upon the development and documentation of clear operational definitions of actual regulatory requirements, cutting that unnecessary fat described above. The "Operational Definitions" strategy tends to reduce overenthusiastic compliance that exceeds actual regulatory expectations.

Chapter 3 suggests that investing in an independent audit, conducted by either an in-house team or outside experts, will save significant "repair" costs and will speed approval of related submissions. In many cases, the audit will actually replace all or part of an FDA visit, reducing lost response time and permitting more effective facility management.

Quality by Design (QbD) is an evolving FDA initiative for automating significant portions of the quality control process. Chapter 4 provides an explanation, and it discusses the ways in which an investment in a QbD system can result in significant regulatory savings.

Chapter 5 presents the concept of outsourcing as a short-term cost-containment strategy. When used effectively, outsourcing can help build internal expertise at the same time it reduces headcount and taps experience and expertise. Excessive outsourcing can, of course, result in long-term loss of efficiency and control; the chapter suggests tactics for walking that fine line.

The wave trend toward electronic (rather than paper) submissions has been growing over the years, now reaching tsunami levels. Electronics submissions can save assembly time and expense, but more importantly can save review time and move a product more rapidly to market. Chapter 6 describes the process and the advantages.

Chapter 7 looks at the most common approach to submission of new products—NDAs, BLAs, and PMAs—to both the FDA and EMEA, and it suggests a simultaneous submission strategy as an alternative to sequential submissions that can save in both the assembly costs and the review times, carrying similar advantages to the electronic submission.

Coping with FDA visits—inspections and investigations—is a significant cost sink. Chapter 8 provides a strategy for controlling those costs by assuming control of the FDA visit, replacing passivity with managerial responsibility.

The final strategy, Risk Assessment, is described in Chapter 9. This strategy allows controlled investment in regulatory issues by providing a mechanism for determining what actions will make a real difference in theareas of FDA and QA responsibility and focus.

And how do these strategies work in the field? Chapter 10 consists of a number of case studies, drawn from all three industries (medical device, biologics, and pharmaceuticals). In real situations (disguised for obvious reasons) the strategies have been tested over time, and the long- and short-term benefits have been estimated.

Chapter 11 summarizes the field results, analyzes the results, and recommends which strategies are likely to be most successful for each industry and for a variety of circumstances. This chapter will provide the regulatory manager or executive with the information necessary to make and informed implementation decision.

As a special topic analysis, Chapter 12 deals with tactics for coping with regulation in times of chaos, generally resulting from major changes in regulatory guidelines and from the transition period as those guidelines are defined.

Chapter 13 reviews the international regulatory scene. While the USFDA and European EMEA tend to dominate, regulatory agencies in many other countries not only control product development and licencing within their boarders but also influence international agencies including the Organisation for Economic Co-operation and Development (OCED) and the World Health Organization (WHO). This chapter provides a clear model of those areas of influence.

Chapter 14, guest written by scholar Ronald Fuqua, provides a summary of the theoretical base of cost-contained regulatory compliance, along with an applicational model for utilization of that theory to manage a pharmaceutical, biologics, or device organization. It bookends the introductory chapter, and provides a basis for the predictions and coming changes highlighted in the next chapter.

Chapter 15, the last chapter, looks to the future, identifying (a) the major trends that are affecting the Food and Drug Administration today and tomorrow and (b) the impact of those trends on the eight strategies that are suggested.

Several of the cases described in Chapter 10 have been developed by friends and colleagues: my thanks to Carl A. Rockburne, Ronald Fuqua, and Arthur Spalding.

We owe it to the public to bring pharmaceuticals, biologics, and medical devices to market at the most affordable price points possible; containing regulatory costs is a small contribution to the debt.

Special thanks are due to three fellow consultants who contributed to this book:

Dr. Ronald Fuqua of the Department of Health Care Management at Clayton State University

Mr. Arthur Spalding, Founding Partner of TAMM Net, Inc., a medical device consulting firm

Mr. Carl A. Rockburne, President of The Rockburne Group, regulatory consultants

Special thanks are due to Mrs. Janine Cahill for her editorial assistance.

SANDY WEINBERG

Atlanta, Georgia
October 2010

CHAPTER 1

CONTROLLING REGULATORY COSTS

1.1 INTRODUCTION

The United States Food and Drug Administration is continuously in a state of dynamic tension, trying to balance two potentially contradictory goals. The agency is charged with assuring the safety and efficacy of pharmaceutical and biologics products, as well as with encouraging public access to those potential cures and treatments. Setting maximal safety standards would screen out all but the conservative products at the expense of public access to alternate products; rapid and broad approval will provide greater access but at the potential compromise of safety. In recent years this tension has been increased by the realization that product cost is a major inhibitor of access and that overly stringent safety standards significantly increase costs.

The same dynamic tension exists in the industry, which has strong altruistic, legal, and financial reasons to take a very conservative stand on safety, but which needs to control costs and hence avoid unnecessary and nonrequired regulatory affairs and compliance actions. Meeting the FDA's stringent requirements assures safety and efficacy; exceeding those same standards adds to cost without improving quality.

The situation is made all the more complex by the purposeful lack of specificity in FDA regulations, guidelines, and requirements. Because the agency is responsible for such a broad range of products produced under varying technologies with differing controls, very tight standards are not possible (or would be counterproductive). Instead the FDA provides general principles; relies on the industry to be self-regulated; and assigns to itself the responsibility of checking, confirming, and approving that self-regulation. A company that eliminates the quality control/quality assurance processes is not in compliance, regardless of product quality; self-regulation is a key principle of operation.

As a result, many companies find themselves imposing regulatory requirements in access of FDA guideline and intent; find themselves expanding submissions evidence in excess of requirements; find themselves adding inefficient post process quality controls; find themselves in a product delay situation, scrambling to retrofit regulatory controls after an FDA audit of their poorly planned internal controls; and

Cost-Contained Regulatory Compliance: For the Pharmaceutical, Biologics, and Medical Device Industries, First Edition. Sandy Weinberg.
© 2011 John Wiley & Sons, Inc. Published 2011 by John Wiley & Sons, Inc.

generally find themselves significantly overspending on regulatory affairs and compliance in a frustrating effort to insulate themselves potential FDA criticism.

These regulatory and compliance overexpenditures fall into eight categories, which in turn lead to eight cost reduction strategies. First, many organizations are unclear on the operational (as opposed to the formal) definitions of actual FDA requirements and regulations. While they understand the written word in guidance documents, they may not have access to the field interpretation of those requirements—that is, access to what is actually expected by FDA investigators and reviewers. The result is often unnecessary or misdirected expensive actions.

Second, many companies take a passive or reactive position to a forthcoming FDA review or visit. Instead of performing their own independent (credible expert) audit, correcting deficiencies, and providing a reviewer or investigator with a report demonstrating compliance, they choose to "roll the dice" and see what the FDA finds. The result is likely to be costly product launch delays, negative publicity, and expensive post hoc corrections.

Third, few organizations are fully aware of the FDA's Quality by Design (QbD) initiative, which can reduce regulatory review times and expenses by building in and documenting quality controls and assurance, rather than restructuring or retesting while a product sits in quarantine awaiting approval and release. QbD reduces the number of submissions required (by using a Design Space concept to define product specification ranges rather than minimums); introduces a Risk Assessment to evaluate the necessity of production modifications; and utilizes a Process Analytical Technology (PAT) approach to automating quality controls.[1]

Fourth, many organizations are using outmoded human resource models to staff up for regulatory projects more effectively outsourced. An IND application specialist, for example, may be the most efficient person to head a new research submissions team, but wouldn't be kept occupied in all but the largest organization. Hiring instead a submissions generalist assures full workforce utilization, but steps away form maximal expertise and efficiency. Using a highly experienced, focused, and expert outsource specialist team not only is more effective but brings a regulatory credibility and familiarity that can save significantly on unnecessary remediation: The expert team knows exactly what is required, and the FDA has confidence in their assurances.

Fifth, the submission areas permit paper or electronic transmission of documents. Use of a proven electronic technology speeds the review process and encourages greater agency cooperation. But many companies lack the expertise to employ electronic submissions systems or, even worse, rely on kludged or modified hyperlink systems that can frustrate reviewers and slow the review process.

Sixth, many companies redundantly submit regulatory documents and rely on auditing visits from both FDA (United States) and EMEA (Europe). While the regulations in place at these two agencies are not identical, there is sufficient overlap to permit development of strategies that will lead to common documents and evidence to satisfy both organizations, significantly reducing costs.

---

[1] Weinberg, S. A Model of Quality by Design (QbD) Implementation in a Pharmaceutical Manufacturing Process, *ISPE Annual Conference*, October 2008.

Seventh, many companies lack experience or fear reprisal standby passively during FDA visits, afraid to exert normal and appropriate managerial control of the process. The most common results of this passivity is suspicion on the part of the FDA, a misunderstanding of roles on both sides, and a lack of productive exchange of recommendations and information.

Finally, too many organizations lack the skills, tools, or expertise to try and prioritize regulatory initiatives, and they find themselves treating all guidelines as equal and applying all recommendations to all situations. Without a risk assessment to provide a rational justification for analysis, time, energy, and dollars are spent in insignificant areas and issues better used where a control makes a real difference.

These sight strategic considerations lead to clear cost reduction recommendations that can maintain product safety (and FDA acceptance of that quality) while improving public access through cost controls. Together they outline a comprehensive strategy for cost reduction in regulatory affairs and compliance.

1.2   CLEAR OPERATIONAL DEFINITIONS

FDA guidelines and regulations tend to be general. This tendency is a result of three factors: the diversity of industry, which encompasses a variety of product types, technologies, and approaches; the expected longevity of new regulations, which generally take two to three years to promulgate (discussion, draft release, comment period, final release) and are intended to have a life expectancy of 10 or more years; and the expertise level of FDA investigators and reviewers, who tend to be well-educated, well-trained, and experienced, and hence, as expected, to use their own skills in interpretation. Regulations such as the Good Manufacturing Practices survive decades (with periodic updating), apply to virtually all kinds of regulated manufacturing, and leave ample room for expert interpretation.

The result is analogous to a blind high jumper: Unable to see exactly where the bar is positioned, the jumper extends just a bit extra to be certain to clear the line. As a result, the bar is "raised" artificially without ever being moved upward. If other jumpers follow suit, the effective result will be norm in excess of the established height: When we are not certain what the FDA really requires, the entire industry jumps just a little higher, and the new raised position becomes the norm that investigators and reviewers grow to expect.

The cost reduction strategy is to base regulatory standards and expectations—in the self-regulation of the organization and perhaps the outsider auditor confirming—not on the vague requirements of the FDA guidelines but on the operational definitions. The real standards as used by the industry and applied by the agency are more difficult to determine but more cost effective to reach. With experience, access to norms established through the industry, and analysis of FDA findings (and 483s), it is possible to develop a strategic operational definition of real-world requirements and, hence, to shave the actual bar to a whisker-width.

Consider the testing of software used in document control to assure compliance with 21 CFR Part 11. How large a data sample should be used for the testing? The original guidance that accompanied the first draft of requirement suggests a sample size of 200. The final document makes no mention of recommended sample size. At least one FDA spokesperson has recommended a sample size of 50 cases.[2] The Center for Professional Advancement course of System Validation proposes a formula for test samples based upon a combination of risk assessment and pathway analysis.[3] Yet an examination of common practices in the field (and general FDA acceptance would lead to a sample size of 10–15 data cases.[4] Without a thorough understanding, most companies are likely to conduct more tests—at greater expense—than is necessary.

Costs can be effectively controlled through operational, practical definitions of actual requirements and through the understanding of those requirements to provide the FDA with assurances of effective self-regulation. That self-regulatory quality assurance will provide confidence in product and data, as well as confidence of conformity with compliance expectations.

1.3   AUDITS

FDA visits can be traumatic events. Scheduled events are generally preceded by weeks of preparation. Unannounced investigations force canceled vacations, rapidly assembled teams, and general paranoia. These unannounced investigations tend to disrupt normal operations, to trigger expensive and often cosmetic preparations and response, and, all too often, to result in a "band-aid" approach to identified problems.

Most FDA investigations follow a "systems approach."[5] The FDA team first asks for an inventory of all systems—functional activities—in place at the facility. A manufacturing facility, for example, may have a warehouse management activity, an inventory control system, a quality testing unit, and so on. In all facilities a quality assurance or control system is required.

The FDA will then select from the list the quality system and one or more additional systems (based on previous issues in a "for cause" investigation; or upon a random selection, or upon the team's observations at other sites). Each of the selected systems will be examined according to the general criteria of the GMPs (GLPs, GCPs, etc.), the organization's own Standard Operating Procedures, and the company's self-regulation. The result of the visit will be a summary report (possibly in the form of a 483 report) recommending or requiring remediation; a scrambling by the organization to add on controls or corrections to implement those remediation; and a great deal of internal strife.

But there is an alternative that is less traumatic, is more effective, and avoids the expensive emergency corrective actions.

Well in advance of any scheduled FDA visit (and in advance of any unanticipated visit) the company implements its own audit program. In what amounts to a

---

[2] AABB Conference 2003.

[3] CFPA System Validation, GAMP Harmonization and PAT, Amsterdam, NE, December 2008.

[4] Based on Tunnell experience with more than 150 validation audits over the past eight years.

[5] FDA now mandates a systems approach to all inspections, but the concept is not fully adopted by field investigators. Some teams may still be following the previous "problem trail" guidelines.

series of mock-FDA audits, all systems are reviewed. Based upon the results of those reviews, a "building quality in" program is designed, replacing expensive emergency responses with cost-controlled quality planning. Once the plan is completed and all significant problems are remediated, a final audit report is generated, filed, and updated periodically.

When the FDA arrives and requests a list of systems, the team is provided not only with the list but also with a highly credible audit report. While there is no de jure guaranteed acceptance of that report, de facto results based on more than 40 audits over the past five years suggest that the FDA team is likely (current record: 43/43) to accept the report, review it, and move on to other visit issues.

The key, of course, lies in the credentials of the auditors. For maximum assurance they should meet three criteria: independence (not reporting to the facility manager; if consultants, fee not based on project result), expertise (education, training, and research credentials), and experience (previous familiarity with similar systems in multiple settings).

A major blood processing industry, for example, found that a series of FDA unannounced visits to their multiple production sites were disrupting operations, generating negative publicity, and (as the sites struggled to implemented patchwork changes) adding significantly to cost. They instead brought in a team of independent auditors who developed specific criteria appropriate to the organization's operations; trained key site managers in those criteria; provided advice as the centers implemented appropriate changes; conducted audits; and issued a comprehensive report summarizing and testifying to appropriate compliance with all regulations and guidelines. As a result, the FDA replaced its unannounced visits with periodic reviews of the audit reports, and the organization significantly reduced its compliance expenses.

1.4   QUALITY BY DESIGN[6]

Quality by Design (QbD) is an FDA initiative specifically designed to reduce regulatory and compliance costs. Conceptually, QbD builds quality into a process rather than adding it on as a more expensive overlayer. The three interactive QbD elements—risk assessment, design space, and process analytical technology—together provide a frame for maximum quality assurance at minimal expense.

Risk assessment refers to an identification of the potential danger of system failure in any of the process phases or parts. The risk assessment is based upon categorization of potential failure as *high risk* (direct impact on human health and safety); *medium risk* (only indirect impact on human health and safety); or *low risk* (remote or no impact on human health and safety). These risk severity levels are further mitigated by probability measures, estimating the likelihood of occurrence of the potential problem. Taken together, the severity and probability risk factors provide a prioritization of oversight and (inversely) a flexibility of control levels: A

---

[6] This section is adapted from an invited presentation to FDA CBER and CDER, October 10, 2008, by Tunnell Consulting, Inc.

low risk factor might lead to only a periodic monitoring of performance and a wide range of acceptable performance levels. In contrast, a high-risk element would result in constant monitoring and tightly defined range of acceptance performance (the design space).

That range of acceptability is related to the design space, an analysis of the detailed design elements and the flexibility of performance of those elements. Much as a statistical analysis may test again a range of .05 or .001, or even a tighter tolerance level, the design space analysis results in the determination of the appropriate tolerance levels of quality controls and system performance.

The monitoring of those controls and elements is defined as process analytical technology (PAT). PAT has two critical elements[7]: continuous (rapid, multiple discrete) monitoring and cybernetic (self-correcting) monitoring. A PAT system has continuous monitoring points built into the process; and whereever practical, those monitoring points can adjust parameters (temperature, pressure, etc.) if they exceed norms.

The norms, and their acceptable ranges, are established by the design space analysis. The control points to be continuously and cybernetically monitored are defined by the risk assessment. Together, these three elements—PAT, design space, and risk assessment—provide a clear operational definition of system quality control and assurance.

That clarity can lower costs in two important ways. First, building QbD into a system is relatively inexpensive because it is conceptually designed into the original system plans. In fact, by determining what issues are low risk, and hence have loose tolerances and require little monitoring, the QbD approach may lower original plan costs. More importantly, though, building in is generally less expensive than adding on: If a QbD analysis results in eliminating the need to rework a system at a later date, savings are likely to be significant.

Second, a well-designed QbD system lowers regulatory costs, since it reduces the number of submissions (within design space tolerances, new amendments are not required), lowers the time required for NDA, ANDA, and BLA reviews[8] by the FDA, and is likely to reduce remediations and changes required. Calculated as more rapid time to market, competitive advantage, and patent life, these savings are likely to be very significant.

1.5 ELECTRONIC SUBMISSIONS

Formal communication with the Food and Drug Administration often involves lengthy and carefully constructed submissions of INDs, Annual Reports, NDS, ANDAs, BLAs, and other critical documents. This submissions process can be cost-controlled in two fundamental ways: (1) through the use of specialized experts

---

[7] A third PAT element, the capability of remote monitoring, permits more cost-effective regulatory audits and monitoring, but isn't directly relevant to this discussion.

[8] See Weinberg, S. *Guidebook of Drug Regulatory Submissions*, John Wiley & Sons, Hoboken, NJ, 2009.

guiding the process and (2) through the utilization of tested, accepted electronic submissions systems.

A major FDA submission is generally preceded by a formal meeting request, with a briefing book. The request and subsequent briefing book identify the key issues to be discussed.[9] The meeting is held, answers are supplied, the agency provides a summary of findings, and the company responds. While these steps seem routine, they are of critical importance: The wording of questions, as well as the wording of the company's response to FDA answers, can translate into millions of dollars and years of effort in the clinical testing process. The use of a specialist with specific experience in meetings, submissions, and the specific FDA division or group can be a significant cost reduction factor.

One Midwestern university-based research organization, for example, recently met with the FDA (neurology) to discuss a forthcoming IND. The briefing book questions, however, were poorly worded, without rationale and requested response, and the research organization did not effectively defend their position in the subsequent meeting. As a result, the FDA panel recommended three additional Phase I and Phase II studies. In their response the organization neglected to request modification or clarification of the FDA recommendation and instead agreed to all suggested studies. The result was an unnecessary delay in the drug development process; the expense of more and more extensive studies than were actually necessary; and a significant decline in the financial value of the organization and its drug patents.

Similarly, a successful electronic submissions system can help to structure the submission itself and can speed the review process. To do so, the system must be proven (with wide use by the industry and maximal experience by the FDA) and effective, coordinately closely with all FDA Electronic Submissions guidelines.[10] The use of such as system, under the management and direction of a team familiar with that system, can both reduce up-front costs and reduce downstream costs related to delayed review and evaluation.

1.6   OUTSOURCING

A well-staffed regulatory and compliance department is critical to maintaining FDA relations, preparing timely and successful submissions, developing and implementing regulatory strategy, assuring product quality and laboratory accuracy, and organizing internal documentation and operating procedures. But what is the cost-effective picture for the regulatory and compliance department?

Unless an organization is generating a sufficient number of submissions to keep specialist teams in meeting requests, IND submissions, NDA.ANDA/BLA submission, supplemental submissions, and compliance audits busy on a continuous basis, the best model consists of a coordinating executive, in-house teams of any of

---

[9] It is recommended that these questions be formatted as an explanation of the action the organization desires, a detailed rationale for that action, and a "does the agency agree?" question.

[10] See www.fda.gov/cder/regulatory/ersr/, FDA Electronic Submissions and Review.

the above areas that do represent a steady work stream, and coordinated outsource teams under the direction of that executive. This hybrid outsource model is necessitated by the highly specialized and critically important skills necessary for the four distinct and unique submissions roles and for the credible auditor role.

Consulting companies have traditionally referred to unbillable time between projects as "on the beach." To determine the cost effectiveness of outsourcing, a research or manufacturing organization can use the same concept. If a specialist in a regulatory or compliance area is needed less than 60% of the time—that is, "on the beach" or submaximally utilized more than 40% of the time—it will prove more cost effective to outsource the activity. In a large organization with generous benefits, that figure may be even lower: One major global manufacturing company found that sourcing was cost effective for any function that wasn't needed more than 75% of the time.

There is another calculation to consider. Increasing head count and using in-house personnel for regulatory and compliance people may not be significantly more expensive than outsourcing in the short term, but the real cost of regulatory action isn't the salary, benefits, and overhead of an employee: It is the much more significant expense represented by the delays of an rejected submission, the bad publicity of a recall or major citation, the multiple costs of response to an adverse finding, and the added expense of trying to add on required quality controls that should have been built in originally. Using in-house regulatory generalists may be acceptable in the short term, but having experienced, credible specialists in each compliance and submission area can save the real expenses associated with compliance and regulatory affairs problems.

1.7 EMEA COORDINATION

Harmonization between FDA and European EMEA regulations and policies is primitive at best. The key EMEA document is the GAMP4[11]; the rough equivalent is the FDA's GMPs plus 21 CFR Part 11. While these sets of documents overlap to a large degree, there are important differences in philosophy, approach, and detail that often result in US companies building separate and distinct FDA and EMEA regulatory teams. It is possible, however, to reconcile the differences and develop a number of common tools for meeting the requirements of both regulatory bodies.

In the case of submissions, the conceptual key is to organize data into logical units representing statements and supporting evidence. Those statement units can then be manipulated and organized to represent the responses to the questions framed by the two regulatory agencies. While separate electronic submissions protocols will be required, the logical units themselves will, with proper organization, generally suffice for both agencies.

For regulatory compliance, the FDA's new "systems inspection" initiative closely parallels the EMEA's less confrontational approach. By inventorying all systems in place in a facility (focusing primarily on the self-regulatory nature of the

---

[11] Soon to be replaced with a minor revision, GAMP5.

quality system) and by using independent audit reports or internal audit findings to support the functional control of those unites, the same evidentiary files can be used to meet the requirements of both the European EMEA and the American FDA.

In short, since the post-philosophical differences between the agencies are largely structural and organizational rather than conceptual, it is possible and practical to prepare for inspections and to write submissions with significant overlap. Separate activities with largely redundant cost and effort can be replaced with coordinated design.

1.8 FDA VISITS

The FDA generally uses a systems approach to inspections and investigations, permitting and encouraging companies to prepare in advance internal or independent reviews of quality systems and other significant organizations systems. The criteria for these reviews, as well as the actual inspection checklists used by the FDA, are available from the agency and from private publications. With a little research, it is possible and appropriate to anticipate most FDA questions, to prepare clear responses, and to internally check those responses against operational realities.

This approach, coupled with a Standard Operating Procedures for Visits and Inspections, can allow management to effectively assume responsibility for FDA visits. The result is the difference between an unanticipated intrusion and an FDA-controlled review of a self-regulated and well-controlled company. Of course some FDA issues may emerge in that review, and areas of unanticipated focus may arise, but the majority of the regulatory investigation can and should take place in advance of the arrival of FDA officials.

1.9 RISK ASSESSMENT

"A difference, to be a difference, must make a difference." A risk assessment, evaluating the probability and severity of emerging problems, permits focusing quality and regulatory energies on areas of significance. Consider an example drawn from recent Congressional testimony: two factories, located on opposite sides of the street in rural North Carolina, manufacture medical devices. Both use the same software system to track shipments and to potentially recall faulty devices. Both facilities are therefore subject, at least in theory, to the same regulatory requirements for the system validation of their computers to assure managerial control of these recall systems.

But one facility is a manufacturer of highly sensitive pacemakers, which must be tracked to a specific patient and physician. If a recall is necessary—and, for a variety of reasons, that necessity occurs less than rarely—the specific recipient of a unit and his or her physician must be contracted immediately. Lost or inaccurate data are likely to have severe medical consequences.

The other facility punches tongue depressors—wooden sticks—from native pine, sands the rough edges, packages, and ships to medical facilities. The necessity of a recall is hard to image and is a rarity: in such an eventuality, an email to all of the appropriate customers would simply direct that the affected batch of depressors should be discarded and would be replaced. There is little real danger involved.

Should the same effort of computer validation apply to both organizations? Common sense, along with a risk assessment, would lead to a negative conclusion. And, for the depressor company at least, that conclusion would significantly reduce the costs of regulatory compliance.

1.10 SUMMARY

In the struggle to balance pressures to supply the public with access to lifesaving, life-supporting, and life-enhancing products with the pressures to guarantee the safety and efficacy of those products, pharmaceutical and biologics companies have come to realize that the costs associated with drugs represents a major impediment to that access even as efforts to assure and demonstrate that safety can—without careful controls—significantly multiply those expenses. The solution to the dilemma is to adopt the most cost-effective strategies for proving those safety and efficacy issues.

Cost reduction in regulatory affairs and compliance can best be achieved with an eight-part strategy. Good regulatory relations coupled with specific experience and detailed expertise can provide clear operational definitions of actual requirements, avoiding unnecessary "overkill." Independent audits can take control of regulatory visits and assure that quality controls are built in rather than added on as expensive late corrections. The use of Quality by Design can speed review processes, minimize filings, and provide credible monitoring or process variations within range. Well-organized, detailed, and specific submissions, controlled by experienced personnel, using widely recognized electronic filing systems, can avoid costly additional clinical testing and save preparation time and expense. The judicial use of outsourcing can avoid "beach time" and make certain that all aspects of the compliance and regulatory processes are handled with maximal expertise as well as efficiency. By organizing supporting data for submissions and inspections around coordinate EMEA and FDA requirements, overlaps can minimize cost redundancies. Anticipation of and internal management of regulatory inspections can maintain control and place quality assurance appropriately on the organization. And a risk assessment approach can provide a priority criterion that assures investment of regulatory energies proportional to their value.

Together, these eight strategies can effectively control the costs of compliance and regulation and can avoid the significant expenses of unnecessary delays, additional clinical testing requirements, and refilings.

CHAPTER 2

CLEAR OPERATION DEFINITIONS OF REQUIREMENTS

2.1 INTRODUCTION

In addition to avoiding pork products and shellfish (and some other products), Jewish people, who follow the kosher laws, never mix meat and milk in the same meal. The root reason for this prohibition has important implications for regulatory cost containment.

The Torah (Jewish Bible) has a verse (Exodus 19) that translates "You shall not boil the kid in its mother's milk." While the reason is somewhat obscure (it was probably meant to condemn a ritual practice of another tribe), the direction is quite clear: Don't mix the meat of a baby goat with the milk of its mother.

But early interpreters of the verse wanted to avoid all chance of error; after all, God is the ultimate regulatory authority, with even more power than the FDA! So to make certain the original intent was observed, they decided it was better to avoid mixing any goat meat with any female goat's milk, just in case someone inadvertently made an error. And to be doubly certain, why not prohibit mixing *any* meat with *any* milk. And to be triple certain, we eventually have the modern practice of separate plates, separate dishwashing machines, and separate restaurants for dairy and meat meals. As a side note, since these early regulators were unaware of the difference between mammals (bearing milk) and birds (without milk), they included in their prohibition mixing dairy products with chicken and other fowl meats.

This process, known as "building a wall around Torah," works well for followers of kosher laws and has some advantages of religiosity for its adherents. But the practice does continually build higher and higher fences around FDA regulations just to be certain that there is no possible chance of a violation resulting in unnecessary and unproductive expenses for all too many pharmaceutical, device, and biologics companies.

All too many biomedical companies have adopted increasingly onerous self-regulations as a protection against the perceived ambiguity of FDA guidelines. While

Cost-Contained Regulatory Compliance: For the Pharmaceutical, Biologics, and Medical Device Industries, First Edition. Sandy Weinberg.
© 2011 John Wiley & Sons, Inc. Published 2011 by John Wiley & Sons, Inc.

internal calculations may show that a sample of 20 items per batch is sufficient for testing, the lack of a clear standard leads to a decision to test 30—"just to be sure." At a conference the QA manager hears a consultant (a person who charges by the hour and hence has a built-in bias to make operations and procedures more complex) recommend testing 50 items as "an industry standard" and returns home to urge increasing the requirement. That QA Manager then accepts a position and promotion at a company across town, and he or she increases the standard further to 100 units to prevent any possibility of problems (and to cement his reputation for quality improvement), quickly growing the "industry standard." An FDA investigator visits the now 50-unit company and the across-town 100-unit company and then visits a third facility testing only 30 units, and asks "why so few?" Soon we are all victims of this "arms race" of ever-increasing requirements. We've built a wall around the FDA Torah, with even the benefit of feeling more pious.

Ah, you might think, but we do have better quality standards: always increasing, always improving. But every new standard, every "improvement," carries a cost that is ultimately passed on to the consumer (directly, or though insurance or government subsidy, indirectly). And that cost decreases, perhaps slightly (but increasingly, significantly), the access to that drug, device, or biologic. Consumers, insurers, and governments must make decisions about the relative value versus the cost of every product; and as the costs increases, the consumer decides not to fill that prescription, the insurance company decides not to include that drug on its standard list, and the government decides that the treatment cap does not permit its use. The greater-than-needed quality testing decision has precluded some patients from access to the product.

All regulatory decisions represent a careful balance between two competing priorities: (1) the need to assure that the drug, device, or biologic is safe and (2) the need to maximize access to that product. Either extreme is dangerous, as extremes tend to be. We can decide to approve all new products, regardless of safety, and simply provide patients and their health care professionals with information so they can make their own decisions. This maximization of access at the expense of safety is the argument made for the rapid release of experimental drugs for terminal patients; and as recently as 1970, at least one FDA Associate Commissioner recommended it as a general policy. But most of us would want untested or unproven products on the market, fearing the potential negative effects. All a terminal patient needs is a drug with side effects that make the last few months more agonizing.

Alternately, maximizing safety testing to assure that a biologic is completely safe in all possible conditions for all potential patients is likely to be a strategy that leaves some patients in need of help waiting for years for results of redundant or obscure tests. The complexity of drugs, devices, and biologics, combined with the complexities and diversities of the human body, assure a steady stream of side effects, anomalous reactions, and idiosyncratic responses that arguably mean that no product is universally safe and effective. Every medical student in a pharmacology class quickly learns that the test answer to every question on drug side effects is "possible dry mouth, nausea, diarrhea, and the opposite to the intended reaction"—

there is always someone who reacts to a blood-pressure-lowering drug with raised blood pressure.

The answer, of course, is moderation—no doubt in most everything in life, and certainly in regulation. Balancing the access and safety of a product is (a) the appropriate macro public policy for the FDA and (b) the appropriate micro corporate strategy for the regulatory affairs department. But building an unnecessary wall around a guideline upsets that balance, sacrificing valuable access for ineffective safety precautions. The problem can be avoided, of course, by cost-containing the regulatory procedures. And the key to that cost-containment is finding a clear, unambiguous definition of exactly what is required.

2.2   OPERATIONAL DEFINITIONS

Regulatory definitions of specific requirements are designed to cover a wide range of widely varying conditions. The same definitional guideline may cover (a) a medical device company making wooden tongue depressors and implanted pacemakers, (b) highly dangerous drugs with very narrow dosage bands and more benign pharmaceuticals with much more forgiving dose restrictions, and (c) biologics with critical purity requirements and autologous blood products in which contamination issues have been all but suppressed.

This varying of conditions with standardization of definitions leaves the regulatory agency with two general choices. With the first choice, you can provide very specific standards that may prove inappropriate in some conditions. This is the choice made or forced upon a number of agencies, resulting in the complexity of both (a) Internal Revenue Service (IRS) regulations as every contingent variation is (or is attempted to be) dealt with and (b) regulations by agencies such as the Occupational Safety and Health Administration (OSHA).

A few years ago the author was involved in an OSHA inspection while volunteering as the medical officer at a summer Scout camp. This particular camp had a dining hall overlooking the lake, with a wall consisting of 22 screen doors making up that scenic view. Two of those doors were equipped with lighted exit signs, the others were not.

The OSHA inspector, equipped with a thick volume of very specific definitions of requirements, informed the Camp Director that the remaining 20 doors required lighted exit signs. Since these signs are very expensive, the Director asked if there was any other option. The inspector, checking his book of regulations, suggested that the other alternative was to permanently nail shut all of the extra doors. Such an action would, of course, be significantly less safe, but would meet the letter of the detailed OSHA requirement. (A compromise was reached, and less expensive non-battery signs were installed).

To avoid these kinds of counterproductive situations in which detailed definitions end up forcing ludicrous or inappropriate actions, a regulatory agency has an alternative. Rather than try to write detailed definitions that deal (sometimes awkwardly) with every possible situation, the agency can provide general guidelines that describe principles and leave the detail applications to situational specific interpretations. These general guidelines are the second choice.

The FDA, with its well-designed Good Manufacturing Practices (GMPs), Good Laboratory Practices (GLPs), Good Clinical Practices (GCPs), and Good Tissue Practices (GTPs), has opted for this second strategy. The Good Practices define general principles and leave specific applied operational definitions to the each organization or situation.

The operational definitions must, of course, conform to some basic rules. First, they must be compatible with the relevant Good Practices. If GMPs, for example, call for records of batch and lot number, it is possible to define the format, frequency, or other characteristic of those records, but not to eliminate them completely.

Second, the definitions must be justified. The specific regulations promulgated for a special situation should be tied to industry practices, a generally accepted theory, or some other defensible rationale.

Finally, the definition must be established, reviewed, and approved (by management) prior to its implementation. A post facto definition is always suspect: It is much better to identify the appropriate detailed practice, and then implement that interpretation.

These operational definitions are generally codified and documented in Standard Operating Procedures (SOPs). The GMP batch record-keeping requirement is defined in a SOP that conforms to the appropriate regulation, is in keeping with generally established practices, and is written and approved prior to implementation.[1]

When properly written and utilized, SOPs provide the operational definitions that add the necessary specificity to general requirements and guidelines. A GMP requirement, for example, might call for validation of a manufacturing process. The methodology to be used, size of sample to be employed, and specific testing standard to serve as a cutoff are all specified in the Validation SOP.

Visiting regulators will generally begin by reviewing SOPs. As long as the SOP meets the three tests of general conformity to the regulation (i.e., appropriately validates the process, can be documented to demonstrate reasonable conformity to generally established practices, and predates the actual testing), it is the in-house SOP that becomes the standard for the subsequent inspection. In effect the FDA holds companies to the company's own standard, as long as that standard is appropriate and reasonable and has been established in advance of implementation.

Standard Operating Procedures are used to provide clear operational definitions that direct and fine-tune the general regulatory principles of the GMPs and other FDA requirements. By assuring that those SOPs are appropriate to a specific environment and situation and by avoiding the trap of overreaching those requirements to provide an unneeded buffer, well-written and documented SOPs can significantly help to contain the costs of regulatory compliance.

---

[1] It is, of course, possible to implement a SOP or operational definition to describe a practice in place prior to a new regulation or prior to an organization's effort to conform to that regulation. In such a case the spirit should be preserved by independently developing the SOP and then using it to evaluate or modify the existing practice.

2.3   WRITING COST-CONTAINED STANDARD OPERATING PROCEDURES

The development of effective and limiting SOPs requires a modification in the normal SOP development processes. Traditionally, organizations develop SOPs in one of two general ways. In new organizations and some very structured established organizations, SOPs are developed "top down": Representatives of management, or a team of management and QA people, document the detailed process that line workers are expected to follow. This "top-down" process tends to be very efficient, tends to be relatively easy to develop, avoids the problem of management not approving the procedures outlined in a draft SOP, and tends to very rarely reflect the reality of worker processes. Arguably, most criticisms for "not following SOPs" originate with the top-down approach to development. It is a very rare manager or QA professional who understands the detailed requirements of a specific job.

Several years ago the author was participating in an FDA investigation of an animal testing facility. The inspection team obtained the facility SOPs, which had been top-down developed, to use as the template for evaluation. The SOP in question called for workers to identify a specific rabbit for testing by checking the ear tag and cage label; removing the rabbit from the cage and cradling it in one hand; injecting with the appropriate test material; and returning the rabbit to its cage, rechecking the identification.

Over time, laboratory workers noted that the cage design allowed for injection between the slats of the cage without removal of the rabbit, causing the animals less trauma and reducing the danger of returning a rabbit to the wrong cage. Pushed for time, sensitive to the animal's needs, and careful about their work, the workers evolved a superior methodology that did not conform to the SOP. With a top-down SOP development approach, the result was a Warning of Adverse Finding (483) for nonconformity, even though the new procedure was superior to the documented process.

Aware of the likelihood that workers have greater hands on experience than managers, many organizations use a "bottom-up" development procedure. Line workers describe the actions that they have determined effectively, and they efficiently accomplish their assigned tasks. Managers then review those procedures and approve (or modify) the descriptions, producing a final SOP that conforms to both regulatory guidelines and worker-discovered efficiencies.

While this "bottom-up" procedure is generally superior to the "top-down" methodology,[2] a further modification step is necessary to maximize the cost containment of avoiding overly burdensome processes and repetitions. In the "managerial review" step of the bottom-up approach, efficient managers compare recommended procedures to the actual FDA requirement and guideline and, with the help of their own experience or a consultant's input, to standards utilized by other organizations. The goal is to (a) pare the effort required to the actual minimum and (b) raise the

---

[2]The exception is the development of initial SOPs for a new procedure or organization. In such a circumstance a "top-down" methodology is appropriate, to be followed by a review and possible "bottom-up" revision after a few months of experience.

bar to meet other company (nonregulatory) requirements until a reasonable and defensible level of effort is defined.

Note that the there may be times when the minimalist approach is appropriate, but there may be other circumstances when corporate regulatory history and experience, the particularly sensitive nature of a patient population, or other factors may require high levels of control. Knowing the minimum allows cost-contained control, but it does not necessitate always selecting that least expensive option.

Finally, after the management team has recommended procedural modifications to reflect the actual requirements and industry standards for a testing, validation, review, or analysis procedure, the prudent manager might write a memo explaining and referencing that decision. The memo, again predating the actual implementation of the SOP, can be used to answer the FDA investigator's question of "Why did you decide upon this standard?" Demonstrating that the decision was well-researched and well-reasoned and not simply an arbitrary attempt to save effort goes a long way toward regulatory acceptance.

2.4 EXAMPLE: COMPLIANCE WITH 21 CFR PART 11 IN A QA LABORATORY

The recent regulation 21 CFR Part 11 applies to most computer systems used in a pharmaceutical, biologics, or medical device company and has been widely and consistently interpreted in Laboratory Information Management Systems (LIMS) used to collect and analyze testing data in a quality assurance laboratory.

The document *Guidance for Industry: Part 11, Electronic Records; Electronic Signature—Scope and Application* (August 2003), provides a general, conceptual definition of the required validation of computer systems (Part 11 paragraph 11.30) and refers to predicate rule document 21 CFR 820.70(i), which in turn provides a general description of validation, which reads:

Automated Processes. When computers or automated data processing systems are used as part of production or the quality system, the manufacturer shall validate computer software for its intended use according to an established protocol. All software changes shall be validated before approval and issuance. These validation activities and results shall be documented.

While this paragraph clearly provides a mandate for validating a QA laboratory system (or any other system in use), it does not answer key questions of how, to what extent, how frequently, or to what level of standard. To establish those answers, a regulated company has three choices: the ostrich approach, the cuckoo approach, and the eagle approach.

The ostrich (at least in popular mythology) buries its head in the sand and hopes for the best. Analogously, an organization can wait for an FDA visit (hoping it never comes) and, if inspected and cited, use the adverse finding as a guideline for future action. This approach has two major weaknesses: First, the adverse warning is likely to delay approvals, generates additional inspections, leads to adverse publicity, and negatively affects careers. Second, the 483 adverse warning statement may be too vague to give any real guidance for future action, leaving the ostrich company just as vulnerable in the future to other, inevitable follow-up visits.

The cuckoo (again, at least in legend) lays its eggs in another bird's nest. Similarly, one option for a company is to determine what other companies are doing and then adopt or expand upon their strategies. By attending conferences, hiring managers from other organizations, and reviewing journal articles, it is possible to build a composite picture of how other organizations are interpreting the regulation and, hence, to define an "industry standard." The problem with this strategy, of course, is the "wall around the Torah" problem discussed previously. Every organization adds (or at least claims it adds) a little more effort to make certain it is compliant. Soon, we are all adhering to an artificial industry standard in excess of, and much more costly than, the intent of the original guideline.

While other birds fly, the eagle (at least in popular image and the dreams of Boy Scouts) soars. The final strategy meets that lofty image, while swooping in a power dive to a minimal level of actual application. The eagle strategy calls for a careful analysis of a definition of the regulatory requirement—in this case, system validation as appropriate to a specific setting. That affirmative decision is in effect the process of writing your own requirement. That requirement should be justified [by theory, by reference to government documents, or by expert opinion (a "regulatory finding")] and should be reviewed and approved by the independent Quality Assurance department and by management in advance of application.

For example, an organization might determine that the validation of systems in their environment should follow this general (template) checklist:

CHECKLIST: VALIDATION

Electronic Records—Electronic Signatures

☐ System is used in support of drug-related research, laboratory analysis, clinical research, manufacturing, production, and/or tracking.

☐ Record and/or signature system has been subjected to an appropriate and through system validation audit.

- ▪ Audit conducted within 24 months
- ▪ Audit conducted by independent or outside expert
- ▪ Audit included review of:
  - ○ Testing documentation
  - ○ Development documentation
  - ○ SOP documentation
    - ▪ Change control
    - ▪ Archive
    - ▪ Disaster recovery
    - ▪ Use
    - ▪ Training
    - ▪ Audit trail review
  - ○ Archive
- ▪ Audit included inspection of operating environment

☐ System validation documentation has been collected, including evidence of requirements and design approvals, testing, and implementation.

- ▪ Validation protocol
- ▪ Validation team credentials
- ▪ Development documentation
  - ○ Requirements/design document
  - ○ Trace matrix
- ▪ Standard operating procedures
  - ○ Use
  - ○ Training
  - ○ Change control
  - ○ Archive
  - ○ Disaster recovery
  - ○ Audit trail review
- ▪ Testing
  - ○ Boarder cases
  - ○ Norm cases
  - ○ Code review
- ▪ System inventory
  - ○ Hardware
  - ○ Software

☐ Records are retained for appropriate length of time (generally 10 years or two generations over treatment duration) in machine-readable form.

☐ Records are retained for appropriate length of time (generally 10 years or two generations over treatment duration) in human-readable form.

☐ Records are retained in heatproof, fireproof, flood-protected environment; are appropriately labeled; and can be restored in reasonable (generally 72 hours) time.

☐ Procedures are in place to restrict access to data and records to appropriately authorized persons.

☐ Operations checks of system have been designed in to assure appropriate functioning of hardware and software

☐ Audit Trails (preferable electronic and protected; alternately manual and carefully monitored) have been built into the system to detect and identify data changed, including tracking of time an date of change, change agent; and reason for authorized change

☐ Electronic signatures are utilized only in systems with dual level unique identifier authorizations

  ■ Password/password

  ■ Password/key

  ■ Password/biological

  ■ Other:

☐ Electronic signatures are utilized only in systems with internal procedures to assure that approved documents have not been modified (without authorization) from specified date and time.

  ■ Time system

    ○ Zulu time

    ○ GMT time

    ○ Location-affixed time

    ○ Single time zone

  ■ Date system

    ○ International (dd/mm/yy)

    ○ United States (mm/dd/yy)

☐ A methodology has been implemented to assure the validity of input data. Such methodologies might include dual confirmation of input, the use of check digits, internal norm confirmations, or other techniques.

☐ Systems users and administrators have received appropriate regulatory and functional training.

☐ System users and administrators have ready and constant access to appropriately comprehensive, clear, applicable, timely, and management-approved standard operating procedures (SOPs).

☐ All aspects of the electronic records and electronic signature systems in place have been designed to provide a level of security and control equal to or exceeding the equivalent controls inherent to manual (paper) systems.

Using this checklist (reviewed and approved by QA and management prior to implementation), the organization can then develop and adopt a SOP for validation.

**TITLE: STANDARD OPERATING PROCEDURE FOR
SOFTWARE VALIDATION**

SOP NUMBER: *Draft 0.1*

ISSUE DATE:

EFFECTIVE DATE:

SUPERSEDES NUMBER:

Authorizing Signatures and Date:

I. PURPOSE

The purpose of this procedure is to assure the operation and management of all computer systems and software at a level of control. It will commensurate with all other subcomponents of the manufacturing (GMP) and laboratory (GLP) processes by:

A. Categorizing all systems, subsystems and software components according to the risk to health and safety represented by utilization of that system, subsystem or component.

B. Establishing appropriate levels of control, testing, and documentation for each risk-based category of system, subsystem, or component.

C. Outlining the specific steps to be followed in demonstrating the established appropriate levels of control, testing, and documentation for each risk-based category of system, subsystem, or component.

II. SCOPE

This procedure applies to all computer systems, subsystems, and software components in use with the exceptions of systems that are entirely self-contained and dedicated to:

A. Financial reporting, management and control.

B. Human resource reporting, management and control.

III. REFERENCE

A. August 28, 2002 FDA Letter "Risk-Based Analysis"

B. December 2, 2002 FDA Guideline Document "Determination of Intended Use for 510(k) Devices"

IV. PROCEDURE

A. Categorization

1. Inventory all affected systems, subsystems, and components.
2. Conduct a Risk Analysis for each system, subsystem, or component in accordance with the process outlined in the Safe Medical Devices Act to classify that system, subsystem, or component as:

a. *High Risk*: System failure has low probability to directly and significantly result in an adverse affect on human health or safety (i.e., failure could potentially result in patient death or serious injury or illness.), *or* system failure has high probability to directly adversely affect human health or safety (i.e., failure is likely to result in patient minor injury or illness).

b. *Medium Risk*: System failure has low probability to indirectly result in an adverse affect on human health or safety (i.e., failure could potentially create a situation indirectly resulting in patient death or serious injury or illness.), *or* system failure has high probability to indirectly adversely affect human health or safety (i.e., failure is likely to result in contributing to a situation that indirectly adversely affects human health or safety or failure is likely to contribute to a situation that could in combination result in patient minor injury or illness).

c. *Low Risk*: System failure has low or negligible probability of directly or indirectly resulting in an adverse affect of human health or safety (i.e., failure is not likely to have any adverse patient affect).

(**Note**: Default border cases to next higher level: B to A, C to B.)

3. Determine the risk levels in accordance to the definitions above (2) by:

a. Identifying the adverse system actions through the following:

   i.   Review of historical record.

   ii. Consideration of FDA adverse reaction reporting guidelines (COSTART).

   iii. Analysis of effect of erroneous system decisions and/or classifications.

b. Identifying each of the adverse system actions which determine the probability of that problem by through the following:

   i.   Review of historical records.

   ii. Review of reporting literature (483s and equivalent).

c. Identifying each of the adverse reactions that determine the severity of the adverse event using the following definitions:

   i.   *High severe:* Results in loss of human life; results in major or permanent disability.

   ii. *Medium severe:* Results in nonmajor or nonpermanent disability or significant disruption of quality of life.

   iii. *Low severe:* Does not result in loss of human life, major or permanent disability, nonmajor or nonpermanent disability, or major disruption of quality of life (minor disruption of quality of life only).

d. Utilizing the following chart to determine the level of risk:

Analysis Results	Risk
One or more high-probability, high-severity adverse events	H
Two or more medium-probability, high-severity adverse events	H
Three or more low-probability, high-severity adverse events	H
Majority of events high probability, medium severity	H
Minority of events high probability, medium severity	M
Majority of events medium probability, medium severity	M
All events low probability, medium severity	M
All events low probability, low severity	L

e. Utilize the definitions above in part 2 to mitigate the conclusions of part 3, thus opting for the higher risk level in cases of uncertainty or border.

B. Establish Standards and Conduct Study

1. Define the *Components of a Comprehensive Validation Study* by:

   a. Building a Trace Matrix by charting the links between a Requirements Document, a Design Document, and a Test Script.

      i. *Requirements Document:* Specification of the purposes to which a system, subsystem, or component is utilized.

      ii. *Design Document:* Specification of the features of elements included in the system, subsystem, or component utilized to accomplish the established requirements.

      iii. *Test Script:* Definition of a series of input or process steps with the expected outcome of those steps.

   b. Conducting the System Test(s) in accordance with the Test Script, reconciling any unexpected result through a system correction/retest, test correction/retest, or procedure repetition. Test Scripts must exercise and test each requirement linked on the Trace Matrix. Test Scripts must test general (typical) datasets as well as border condition (variance) data sets.

   c. Reviewing the System Source Code to determine the organizational pattern of the code, the capacities and limitations of the code, and the structure of the code.

   d. Reviewing the User Standard Operating Procedures to assure that procedures conforming to corporate guidelines have been developed, distributed, and implemented to direct:

      i. Normal operations of the system, subsystem, or component

      ii. Problem response

      iii. Change control

      iv. Archiving of electronic and human readable data files

      v. Disaster recovery

      vi. User training

      vii. Electronic signature (if applicable)

      viii. System audit

   e. Conducting a system, subsystem, or component Installation Qualification (IQ) upon first implementation of the system, documenting an appropriate installation and initial function test.

   f. Conducting a system, subsystem, or component Operational Qualification (OQ) of the system pending initial use and documenting appropriate controls and utilization.

   g. Conducting a system, subsystem, or component Performance Qualification (PQ) reviewing error or performance logs, the system audit trail, and general operations, thus documenting appropriate ongoing controls.

   h. Auditing the system vendor or developer via live visit, questionnaire, third-party review, or equivalent mechanism to determine vendor/developer's ability to track and notify in the event of significant error discovery. Then to support and maintain system, subsystem, or component and to maintain appropriate developmental documentation sufficient to augment error response.

2. For all classified systems, subsystems, or components:

a. *High Risk*: Complete all the requirements to define the components of a Comprehensive Validation Study.

b. *Medium Risk*: Complete only the requirements a, b, d, e, and h to define the components of a Comprehensive Validation Study.

c. *Low Risk*: Complete only requirements e and h to define the components of a Comprehensive Validation Study.

Note that this SOP not only is designed to provide a clear definition of requirements, eliminating ambiguity, but also utilizes a Risk Assessment concept to further limit regulatory costs. While this SOP is certainly not a mandatory outline or format and can be extensively modified to meet company standards and need, it does serve to illustrate principle. The eagle approach of proactive definition places the organization in the position of clearly defining and limiting responsibility in areas where the FDA, appropriately, has left room for interpretation.

2.5 RISK ASSESSMENT

As the SOP template (above) demonstrates, the strategy of establishing internal regulatory operational definitions of standards carries with it another significant advantage: The FDA permits and encourages the use of a Risk Assessment as a part of the definitional process.

A Risk Assessment evaluates the likelihood and potential severity of significant risky outcomes, and it uses that analysis to place the situation into crude categories of "high," "medium," and "low" risk. In a manufacturing facility, for example, the use of an air scrubbing system may result in a classification of airborne contaminants as "low risk." In a blood processing operation, the use of patient reports of possible viral exposure may classify that environment as "high risk." The categories are broad and require specific definition for each particular case, all based upon the probability and severity of potential life-threatening problems.

Once a mechanism for determining high-, medium-, and low-risk situations has been defined (with border cases defaulting to the higher category), it is possible to assign varying levels of testing, validation, and control based upon the risk level. In effect, the approach allows spending less time, energy, and investment on controlling risks that are not significant. Most often a three-tier operational definition and SOP is utilized, providing separate standards for high, medium, and low risks.

Because most risks are remote and unlikely and because many regulatory environments include secondary checks and safeguards, many situations are appropriate defined as "low risk" or "medium risk." And the use of less rigorous standards of control for these situations can result in significant cost savings while maintaining regulatory compliance and product/patient safety.

2.6 SUMMARY

Imagine the role of regulator visiting your pharmaceutical, biologic, or device site. The job is overwhelming. If you are a representative of the EMEA, Japanese Ministry, or other non-US agency, it is likely that English (or at least American English) is not your first language; despite your degree of fluency, you must constantly be on the lookout for subtle nuances of language, unique idioms, and cultural variations in interview, documents, and even casual conversations.

If you represent the FDA, you are probably treated with deference tinged with suspicion. In many organizations there is an underlying belligerence—in all, a feeling that a misstep may result in embarrassing legal actions.

You are expected to be an expert while the technology is likely to be unique and the applicational area is likely to be tightly focused and obscure. The home office is pressing you to move as rapidly as possible despite a near overwhelming volume of documents, and an attorney and regulatory representative from the company appear ready to pounce if you miss any section or confuse any finding. And your regulatory guidelines—with which you are expertly familiar—are often vague, sometimes self-contradicting. The potential to end up feeling like a fool is high; the pressure not to is intense.

Imagine, too, the relief you feel when the visited company is well-organized and presents for your review a series of clearly documented, internally reviewed, signed, and dated (prior to testing) specific standards. Each SOP is tied to the appropriate legal regulation; each interpretation has an explanation that is footnoted to an expert opinion, regulatory guideline, or other credible source. And the internal SOPs demonstrate a clear understanding of, and respect for, the principles of patient and product safety.

Your task is now clearly defined: to review and either accept or take specific issue with the operational definitions of the applicable regulations and to review the evidence supplied in support of conformity to those definitions. Both tasks are manageable, are appropriate to your training and experience, are not dependent upon a detailed understanding of the product chemistry, engineering, or design, and will result in reasonable assurance of regulatory compliance and ultimate control (or will clearly identify weaknesses and problem areas).

The responsibility has been appropriately placed with the situational experts, and the regulatory investigator is, as intended, cast in the role of determining whether and to what degree the regulated company has taken responsibility for their own quality assurance.

The cost of compliance has been contained through the judicial use of clear, operational definitions of real regulatory requirements, and the risk is mitigated and is not dependent on the inflationary effect of building higher and stronger walls in an attempt to understand the whims and future preferences of a higher power.

CHAPTER 3

PREREGULATORY AUDITS

3.1 INTRODUCTION

In part due to the complexity of the industry, and in part due to the budgetary and expertise limitations of the agency, the United States Food and Drug Administration classifies the pharmaceutical, biologics, and medical devices industries as "self-regulated." It is the agency's task to oversee and assure the regulation, but primary responsibility for the oversight of quality rests with the industry itself. It is as a direct result of this important distinction that a company without an implemented quality oversight plan is out of compliance, even if the actual formulation and manufacturing procedures meet established standards. To be in compliance, a company must develop and manage a quality control and assurance process in oversight of its discovery, development, manufacturing, or distribution procedures.

In typical operation, then, a pharmaceutical, biologics, or device company establishes its procedures (documented as Standard Operating Procedures), and it includes key quality control points to assure product purity and safety. Prior to packaging or distribution, the company conducts its own in-house Quality Assurance check, thereby reviewing the quality control results, sampling the final product review to be certain that SOPs were rigorously followed, and resolving any questionable or cloudy issues.

On an irregular basis an FDA team may arrive at the front door to conduct an unannounced inspection. This visit generally focuses on a detailed review of the quality assurance and control system, and possibly additional reviews of randomly or purposefully selected other systems. The redundancy of reviews—in-house and FDA—is designed to confirm the ongoing operation of a sound internal quality assurance and control system.

By statute the FDA is directed to visit every site every two years; but in practice, agency-limited resources have modified that norm: Gaps between visits of four years or more are not unusual. And should an FDA visitation team find a major problem, the assumption is made until disproved that that problem dates to immediately after the previous inspection; while unusual, it is possible that a significant issue could trigger a recall of all product manufacturer over the previous four years. Perhaps more important, such a finding could open a four-year window of liability for product shipped under questionable quality controls.

Cost-Contained Regulatory Compliance: For the Pharmaceutical, Biologics, and Medical Device Industries, First Edition. Sandy Weinberg.
© 2011 John Wiley & Sons, Inc. Published 2011 by John Wiley & Sons, Inc.

Added to this potential window of liability problem is a complication of agency expertise. Even the most experienced investigator is likely to have focused areas of expertise, leaving knowledge gaps. The expertise of FDA investigators is complicated by two competing phenomena. First, the agency, which grew exponentially in the 1960s and 1970s, is now graying. As experienced field investigators are reaching retirement years, they are being replaced with younger, less experienced agents. The effect is a loss of experience and an increased likelihood that a visiting team will be dominated by persons who may not have seen that kind of system or product previously.

The situation is further complicated by the parallel problem of increasing complex discovery, development, and manufacturing processes. Computerized, process analytical technology-based, quality-by-design procedures and increasingly multistep chemical processes call for greater and greater industry expertise. But an FDA investigator is broadly trained and is unlikely (all the more so if inexperienced) to understand the complexities of a broad spectrum of modern operations. Arguably the entire industry is becoming one of specialists, lacking the detailed understanding that would allow anyone to operate with confidence in traditional pharmaceutical, device, and biologics environments. Yet it is this breadth that is assumed and required of FDA investigators.

It is this very problem of increasing breadth and decreasing depth that has led the FDA to the "self-regulated" designation: The agency focuses its agents upon the content of the regulations and guidelines and on the analysis of quality systems. But understanding some issues may transcend mastery of regulations and of quality systems and may fall beyond the limited experience scope of an investigatory team. In such circumstances the FDA must make an assumption beyond their understanding, demand controls potentially in excess of situational norms, act upon incomplete knowledge, or trust the actions of the very companies they are regulated. The result is unlikely to be to the benefit of any party: the agency, the company, or the public.

The alternative to this flawed model of in-house QA/QC and external (but with limited experience and expertise) FDA oversight is the addition of a third party to the process. This third party must have (a) the confidence of the FDA, (b) sufficient expertise and experience to understand the detailed environment and processes, and (c) sufficient independence to offer a real and effective check on internal QA/QC systems.

In addition to improving the effectiveness of the quality oversight process, the use of an independent, expert, credentialed outside auditor has four cost-containment advantages: (a) reduction of liability, (b) avoidance of unnecessary quality controls dictated by misunderstanding, (c) immediate correction of a problem, and (d) planned rather than patchwork interventions.

The liability is a direct result of the potential and likely delay between FDA visits. Should an inspection find a problem without a specific and definable start date—for example, a procedure and lack of a control that was not a standard practice at the time of a previous visit—an adverse finding might appropriately throw suspicion on all products produced and shipped over a two-, three-, or four-year period. These batches may be identified as potentially substandard, contaminated, mislabeled, or misformulated. The company may incur some consumer liability, but at the very least would be forced to bare the cost of negative publicity of a major product recall.

An additional expense may result from limited understanding by FDA personnel of the appropriate quality controls for a product. For example, latex condoms are generally subject to two leak tests: (1) a rigorous water test on a sample of condoms and (2) a less accurate spark test on all condoms.[1] A (European) manufacturer of a new design of plastic condoms developed a technique of nondestructive water testing of all of their condoms, and therefore it eliminated the less accurate spark test. Until expert intervention explained the situation, the USFDA was prepared to demand both the (unnecessary) spark test and the more accurate water test (on at least a sample of devices). The FDA's lack of expertise would have resulted in significant increased costs without quality value.

When a problem occurs, the most cost-effective general strategy is to quickly identify and eliminate the difficulty. Waiting to see if the problem will pass regulatory muster adds expense and potential product danger. Product is wasted and must be discarded, discounted, or recycled; recalls can be expensive; and fixes often require a halt in and reworking of production lines. Waiting for an FDA visit rather than quickly detecting and responding to a product is a costly and inefficient strategy.

Finally, responding to the problems identified by often inexperienced and inexpert FDA investigators with patches to the found problems, rather than comprehensive understanding of any system difficulties and implementation of a comprehensive solution, is a costly proposition. While patches tend to solve immediate problems, they tend to create weaknesses of their own. All too often the next round of inspections finds problems with the patches implemented to correct the past problems, and so forth. A comprehensive analysis conducted independently and with real expertise is likely to result in a less expensive and more effective long-term solution.

Thus the addition to the "internal QA/QC plus sporadic FDA oversight investigations" model of an independent expert auditor whose report will provide management with a comprehensive corrective strategy and will provide the FDA with a clear and credible audit report. It is a valuable cost-containing compliance strategy. Implementing that strategy carries real advantages when the auditor brings expert credentials to the table.

3.2 AUDITOR CRITERIA

In order to serve in an effective and credible intermediary quality role, standing between the company and the FDA, an auditor must meet a nebulous but important series of criteria. Philosophically, the auditor must be perceived by the future visiting

---

[1] Latex condoms are manufactured by dipping a steel mold in liquid latex. A spark is then applied to the mold; if the latex is intact, the spark is insulated and the condom is rolled off the mold for packaging. Samples of the packaged condoms are then selected and filled with water under pressure. These selected condoms are discarded after testing.

FDA team as independent, expert, experienced, and credible. Operationally defining these characteristics is problematic at best.

There are some clear disqualifications. While the auditor can be from the same company to be audited ("internal") or from outside the company ("external"), the reporting relationship of the auditor must be completely separate from the organizational unit to be audited. That is, an auditor may be a member of the company, but only if he or she reports outside the chain of command of the audited division. Similarly, because the auditor is in fact evaluating the quality assurance and control system, the auditors reporting the relationship must be outside of the QA/QC group.

An external auditor must be compensated with a prenegotiated flat fee, not a contingency or hour rate that might cause the auditor financial benefit or harm if problems are ignored or exaggerated. And the role of the auditor is distinct from that of a consultant: If the same person or organization both finds and is paid to correct a problem, independence is compromised.

The experience requirement is trifold: An effective auditor should have prior experience (presumably as a junior member of a previous audit team) with the type of product manufactured or development; with the process or procedure in use; and with the quality assurance/quality control roles. That experience should ideally be both broad (exposure to a variety of products, systems, and quality designs) and deep (involving intensive review of management of at least some of those systems).

Expertise is established through a combination of academic achievement, industry training, and auditor authorship of referred papers, articles, and books. While there are no set standards for the level of expertise required, generally the higher the expertise, the more credible the audit.

An independent, experienced, expert auditor should append his or her resume to the final audit report. That resume will be carefully reviewed by the FDA field investigator to determine the credibility of the report. Of course, if the auditor is known to the investigator either through prior contact or reputation, the credibility of the report is enhanced and is de facto established.

Finally, the audit procedure must be established with a clear Standard Operating Procedure approved in advance of the audit. The SOP generally includes checklist or description of the audit points to be included. A credentialed, credible and independent auditor following a preestablished audit SOP provides the most effective and useful intermediary role. While it is not an established FDA policy, the field investigator will generally review such an audit report rather than conduct a detailed inspection and is likely to defer to the opinion of the knowledgeable expert.

3.3 ADVANTAGES OF AN INDEPENDENT AUDITOR

The use of a credible independent auditor is not a regulatory requirement and may at first look appear to be an added expense rather than a cost containment strategy. But an auditor carries two distinct advantages that may significantly reduce the cost of regulatory compliance in a pharmaceutical, device, or biologics organization.

First, the auditor is, by definition, unofficial. All findings by the US FDA are subject to the Freedom of Information Act, and hence are available to the public. A number of industry newsletters, blogs, and media sources have filed open FIA requests and publish all adverse findings (483s). A finding by an independent auditor is not public, however, and is seen only by management.

This privacy not only avoids public embarrassment but also provides another opportunity for correction. In a non-auditor model, problems may be identified by the subject department itself and corrected privately, and/or they may be identified by the QA/QC department, and corrected without external display. On the other hand, a subsequent FDA visit that identifies additional problems will rapidly find itself into the press. An auditor can observe a problem, call for its correction, and then re-audit, so the final report only shows (presumably) problem-free findings.

The private nature of the audit is likely to be less intimidating to the organization's employees and culture, and less disruptive of normal operations. And because that pressure is removed, employees are likely to be more candid about procedures and activities. All employees should be carefully trained to answer FDA questions truthfully and accurately. With an outside auditor, however, that honesty is supplemented by the volunteering of additional information beyond the narrow limits of a specific question. The result is a more thorough and accurate picture than that obtained by an FDA investigator.

The private nature of the audit also affects the scheduling of the event. An FDA visit is scheduled at the convenience of the agency; it does not account for vacation schedules, production plans, quarterly reports, or other events that may have an influence upon the smooth running of the rest of the organization or its employees. An independent audit is scheduled at the convenience of the company. The auditor works around the company calendar, thereby minimizing disruption and interference.

The second advantage of an independent auditor is potentially even more valuable: An experienced and expert auditor has the depth of understanding that can further reduce disruption, can more accurately assess potential problems, and can cope with cultural and linguistic problems.

Because an auditor is a specialist, hired or assigned because of real understanding of the processes or environment in question, there is likely to be much greater knowledge depth than in the FDA generalist. That knowledge depth can result in (a) a briefer but more thorough investigation, reducing disruption time without a loss of detail, (b) a more complete understanding of problem roots and potential corrections, and (c) a rapid grasp of problem subtleties that may be beyond the understanding of the FDA investigator.

In addition, it is likely that the auditor is a "repeater." An internal auditor may revisit a particular system or process on an annual basis; an outside auditor may be re-retained every year or two to update audit findings. With repeat visits comes a further depth of understanding as the auditor observes improvements and does not need to reconstruct a foundation knowledge base. FDA investigators—who visit less frequently, are responsible for a very large number of organizations and products, and are assigned randomly to sites and situations—may find themselves always conducting initial visits (or problem-related follow-ups focusing on very specific issues) but rarely, if ever, get a broad timeline picture of an organization or process.

The added expertise of a specialist, selected because of experience and in-depth understanding of a specific situation and often familiar with that operation from previous visits, can be very effective in finding hidden problems, identifying real solutions, and rejecting inappropriate, expensive, or ineffective work.

There is an old joke about a building manager who is experiencing problems with the boiler that heats his building. He calls an expert plumber, who examines the system, pulls out a piece of chalk, and draws a small "x" on the lower left side of the faulty boiler. The plumber then pulls out a small brass hammer, and gently taps the "x". The boiler immediately returns to ideal performance specifications, and the problem is solved.

A week later the building manager receives a bill for $1000. Outraged, she calls the plumber and demands a breakdown of the charges. The next day he receives a more detailed bill:

Tapping boiler with hammer	$5.00
Knowing where to tap	$995.00

The added expertise of a specialist auditor is likely to result in significant savings of time and trouble because the auditor "knows where to hit."

3.4 COST CONTAINMENT

In many cases the FDA will de facto accept the audit report in lieu of a detailed investigation. The FDA team will, in effect, review the credentials of the audit team and the thoroughness of the report, spot check the findings, and direct their own energies to other (not included in the audit) areas of concern. The audit becomes the primary evidence of "self-regulation," and the audit team will be the arbiter of facility, system, or operational compliance.

The use of independent auditors as an "insurance" intermediary between QA/QC procedures and FDA investigations can result in significant savings and cost containment. These cost containments are a result of three phenomena missing from an ad hoc response to an FDA visit: strategic planning, designed response, and parallel implementation.

At the conclusion of an FDA visit the investigation team provides a written or oral briefing on adverse findings. While an immediate response is not required, many organizations feel pressured to offer on-the-spot corrections, promises of remediation, or rebuttal. Even if the company resists these pressures and (appropriately) responds in a follow-up letter, time is critical: Products or data results produced between the adverse finding and remediation are suspect, and more serious problems may result in a suspension of activity pending correction.

The independent audit eliminates this time pressure, replacing it with an opportunity to examine observations in detail, to determine the extent, significance, and commonality of a finding, to consider alternative fixes, and to implement those fixes in a timely manner. Effectively used, the time and opportunity to plan produced by the independent audit provides cost containments in the form of carefully planning and well-organized response.

That response can be designed into a comprehensive quality system, using the techniques and philosophy of Quality by Design (see Chapter 4). A QbD approach can provide continuous monitoring of key variables and immediate correction of any measures out of specification. But a QbD implementation requires strategic planning: An independent audit can provide the necessary foundation for the planning, and the opportunity to implement.

Finally, the very nature of that implementation can be enhanced as a direct result of an independent audit. Once an audit has identified procedures to be modified, there are two general paths to those corrections. One can use a replacement strategy, discontinuing the inadequate control or inappropriate action; the result is a corrective action that all too often produces its own quality ripples as the replacement procedure is tweaked and toned. Or, in a safer and more cost-effective procedure, the new control is implemented in parallel to the old, testing for problems and tweaking of line until a smooth transition is assured. This parallel implementation is much less likely to be disruptive and is much more likely to result in continuous quality production of pharmaceutical, device, and biologics products.

But parallel implementation requires time, advanced planning, and a designed response—all luxuries provided by an independent audit and all too often lost in the scramble to respond to an FDA investigation.

3.5 SUMMARY

A comprehensive audit, diligently conducted by an independent, expert, experienced, credible audit team, can result in significant savings and cost containment. The small investment for the auditors can result in significant expense offsets because the identified problems are corrected in a planned, organized, and timely manner rather than piecemeal under the pressure of FDA findings. And as the FDA focuses its attention appropriately on the thorough audit report, the independent and planning audit can serve as an insurance policy protecting against errors or misunderstandings from inexperienced or non-expert FDA investigators.

An independent audit is not a requirement; an organization can be in full compliance with ongoing self-controls from QA/QC, awaiting the results of unscheduled FDA investigations. But the audit can help the self-regulated organization maintain control over the FDA investigation as well as the quality process. In doing so, the audit provides an effective cost-containment strategy, permits careful planning and organization in response to an identified problem, and allows senior management a respite from the pressures that a hovering FDA creates.

CHAPTER 4

QUALITY BY DESIGN

4.1 INTRODUCTION

In this era of instant communications, dominated by twitter, email, 24-hour news, and electronic messaging, one media is unique. Unique among almost all other means of recording and communicating information, books stand as the least timely. You are reading these words nine or more months after they are written; rather than timely, a book author must strive for timeless. Bound and published words are intended to carry the virtue of longevity, reflecting truths and opinions that will transcend immediacy.

The result of this pressure to be timeless pushes the author to carefully ponder, edit, and consider every description and prediction. As a result, the work (if successful) carries values of insight, evaluation, and thoughtful contemplation. These advantages, missing in a media in which immediacy is primary and contemplation is an absent luxury, have a tragic limitation. Words crafted during an evolving process are unlikely to reflect the final reality. Writing before concrete decisions have been made, before policies are finalized, and before regulations are established carries the risk of misreport or misinterpretation.

The FDA's "Quality by Design" (QbD) initiative is a prime example of a nebulous, evolving regulatory approach that is just beginning to gel into a key component in regulatory compliance. While QbD has been a prime engineering principle for more than a decade, it has only attracted FDA attention in the last few years. In 2008 this author was invited by the Center for Biologics Evaluation and Research (CBER) and the Center for Drug Evaluation and Research (CDER) of the FDA to present the agency with a workshop defining and describing the processes and advantages of QbD; the results of that workshop and of other presentation and committee efforts are just beginning to evolve into early definitions, guidelines, and proto-regulations.

The tale of four blind men who describe an elephant is apocryphal but potentially serious: One holds the tail and envisions the beast as rope like; another touches the elephant's side and "sees" a wall; a third feels and ear and describes the elephant as very much like a fan; and the fourth holds the trunk and describes a snake. While they are individually thinking about the same animal, their lack of a common understanding of its nature is founded in confusion.

Cost-Contained Regulatory Compliance: For the Pharmaceutical, Biologics, and Medical Device Industries, First Edition. Sandy Weinberg.
© 2011 John Wiley & Sons, Inc. Published 2011 by John Wiley & Sons, Inc.

The first step in understanding any new regulatory initiative is the development of a clear and operational definition of the concept. The operational definition assures that researchers and industry experts are looking at and thinking about the same phenomenon. Without a clear common meaning, terms blur and concepts dissipate into rope–wall–fan–snake arguments.

Over the past three years, the US Food and Drug Administration has introduced the concept of QbD, initially for improving quality assurance and control in pharmaceutical manufacturing.

Yet even at this early stage it is clear that QbD represents an effective and cost-containing strategy for assuring product oversight a minimal monetary and resource allocation. Perhaps more importantly, it is possible even as policy evolves to see the likely shape of the final Quality by Design FDA position and to shape a strategy for cost-contained compliance around that emerging position.

While the engineering concept of QbD is considerably more complex (and rich), the FDA's evolving position is focusing on three major aspects: Process Analytical Control, Design Space, and Risk Analysis. Together, these elements provide a framework for quality assurance and control that is both cost-conserving and end-product quality assuring. While QbD is not likely to be a requirement anytime in the foreseeable future, it is likely to provide an effective optional methodology for providing quality control and assurance at reasonable expense and, hence, will prove an attractive approach for many pharmaceutical, device, and biologics organizations.

Since 2001 the FDA has acknowledged that its carefully balanced, often contradictory responsibilities to assure public access to drug, device, and biologics products and simultaneously to restrict from the market all but the proven safest of those products has resulted in an unintended consequence. Because quality reviews and procedures subtly and overtly influence the economics of production, some (perhaps many) Americans were finding themselves in the unpleasant position of having restricted access based upon ability to pay for life-improving products. Cost was emerging as a significant factor to access, so that as cost-increasing quality controls led (at least hopefully) to increasingly safe products, the same expenses (added to the cost of the products) reduced the number of people who could afford that therapy. In very specific ways, increased safety was reducing access.

The principle in QbD rests in the core definition of "quality." Traditionally, quality is viewed as the absence of defect: no deviation from standards in a medical device; no contaminants, impurities, or infectious agents in a biologic; no variations from content, distribution, and design standards in a pharmaceutical. Quality, in short, was defined as the absence of problems. In a successful system, quality problems were precluded, and there were no flaws that could introduce a potential problem. In somewhat of a logical deviation, any future problems that did creep in could be readily detected.

Quality by Design replaces that "problem-free" definition with a more proactive concept of quality. Quality isn't simply the absence of deviations, impurities, and so on: It is the system itself, constructed to reduce or eliminate the potential for those problems to ever exist in the first place.

Consider, for example, a simplified food warehouse, used for the storage of bags of flour. In a traditional quality scenario, the warehouse could be equipped with traps designed to detect vermin; could be physically screened to minimize entrance by mice, flies, beetles, and so on; and might include a sifting step to remove maggots, insect parts, and so on. The resulting flour on a grocer's shelf would presumably meet quality standards.

In a QbD scenario, the same warehouse would be redesigned, perhaps through the use of negative air pressure, to avoid producing the olfactory clues that would attract vermin, and it would be effectively designed to seal against any incidental invasion. Rather than removing the mouse droppings and insect parts from the finished product before use, the system would be designed to assure that those elements were never introduced at all. The quality controls and assurance checks would be designed in rather than added on to the system. When properly implemented, the result is a seamless environment, effectively sealed against problems as effectively as the warehouse would be sealed against rodents.

This near-miraculous accomplishment, or at least the processes intended to approximate the lofty goal while more mundanely minimizing the traditionally defined quality problems, is the result of three interactive and overlapping elements that together provide a construct model of QbD. QbD presumably provides the highest level of quality assurance and control through the use of (a) a Design Space analysis to identify the variations from norm that constitute potential system threats, (b) the use a Risk Analysis to prioritize those threats, and (c) the implementation of a Process Analytical Technology (PAT) to detect, eliminate, and/or self-correct to avoid those threats.

4.2 QBD FACTORS

Quality by Design has emerged from a confluence of four factors,[1] ultimately leading to the three QbD elements of PAT, Risk, and Design Space. First, process guidelines such as ICH Q8 have matured sufficiently as to define the design space of a process and to identify the input variables and procedures associated with any stage of the research, design, development, production, and distribution process. The ICH guidelines also help to identify the acceptable (and unacceptable) variations of a process and permit the establishment of functional design parameters.

Second, financial and political pressures have stretched the FDA's resources to the point where the agency is actively seeking regulatory streamlining and increasingly accepting the role of oversight agency for a self-regulated industry. In this new scenario the internal quality assurance unit of each organization acts as the primary regulatory enforcement agency, while the FDA assumes an oversight role, checking the performance of the QA units. Such a role requires that the agency define for the industry the specific parameters of self-regulation: QbD promotes that process.

Third, statistical methodologies have evolved to provide empirical interpolation tools that can serve as statistical models with robust predictive power, even

[1] Kamm, J. Can You Win the Space Race? *Pharmaceutical Manufacturing*, May 2007.

when the fundamental principles of a process (such as the function of solids) is not fully understood. In advance of explanatory theory, these statistical models can identify the key variables and their relationships, providing focus for monitoring and ultimately providing the data that theory-building requires.

Finally, the political acceptance of a risk-based approach to regulation, emerging within the FDA since 2001, makes possible the monitoring of process variables without forcing the costs and complexity of trying to measure every conceivable variable in an ever-expanding potential situation.[2] Without this acceptance, the application of statistical tools and regulatory guidelines would create a self-defeating situation swamped in expensive and unnecessary data. With a risk approach, new methodologies can be triaged appropriately.

Together these four factors—sophisticated guidelines, resource pressures, statistical tools, and an acceptance of a risk-based approach—have created a QbD perfect storm. That storm is currently impacting on manufacturing production.

Quality by Design is a conceptualization rapidly gaining traction in the biomedical industries, led by an FDA initiative to reduce costs, increase quality control, and shift the primary responsibility for quality assurance firmly onto the industry. While initially focusing on the manufacturing sector, QbD is increasing, being adopted by automated laboratories. In that laboratory setting, where processes focus on sample control, testing, data collection, data analysis, and decision-making, Process Analytical Technology can provide continuous. cybernetic, and potentially centralized remote monitoring. At the same time, an effective Risk Analysis can define acceptable limits on parameters, prioritize those parameters, and assign appropriate foci on the most important and critical of the measured variables.

4.3 THE MODEL

Quality by Design (QbD) is an initiative of the US Food and Drug Administration and the biomedical industries it regulates, intended to integrate the quality process through research, development, manufacturing and distribution. When properly implemented, QbD improves speed to market, reduces product variation; improves operating efficiency, and reduces costs at all stages of the process. This stochastic model provides an operational definition of QbD in a pharmaceutical manufacturing process and can be used to measure conformity to QbD principles as well as comparative evaluation of QbD systems. Implications of this model include: identification of the significance of Process Analytical Technology and Process Understanding; in-depth analysis of the continuing significance of GMP compliance and conformity with internal Standard Operating Procedures; and in-depth analysis of the relationships of these critical variables (Figure 4.1).

Data for this preliminary stochastic model are drawn from four case studies: one in a QA lab setting, two in manufacturing environments, and one integrating a manufacturing facility with a drug submission.

---

[2] Weinberg, S. Early Warning: Attitude Adjustment at FDA, *American Biotechnology Laboratory*, July 2003.

[QbD] = ((PATcyb + PATmon)/2) + UP + R)/3) ∗ (1/ΔGMP) ∗ (1/ΔSOP)

QbD = conformity with FDA Quality by Design Initiative

PATcyb = Process Analytical technology cybernetic (self-correcting) capability

PATmon = Process Analytical Technology continuous monitoring of critical variables

UP = Measurement of the depth and extent of understanding of the process and the associated design space

R = measurement of the result of a Risk Assessment, assigning priority to functional areas most closely associated with health and safety issues

ΔGMP = variance from conformity of general operating controls with current Good Manufacturing Practice regulations

ΔSOP = variance from conformity with functional Standard Operating Procedures in place in the facility

Figure 4.1

The next steps include tweaking the model based upon a larger data set and then testing the predictive power of the model.

Quality by Design has three key elements: Risk, Design Space, and Process Analytical Technology monitoring. Risk refers to the assessment of relative impact of each fundamental part of a process on human health and safety. It is generally characterized (rather crudely) as high (direct impact), medium (indirect but significant impact), or low (insignificant impact) and is represented in the model by the "R" variable.

The Design Space measures the multi-dimensional region of flexible conformity to established standards: the range within which a variable's values are considered acceptable. In the model, the Design Space is represented by "UP," the measurement of the depth of understanding of the process and the associated design space. The better a process is understood, and the greater to which the range of accepted values have been successfully tested, the higher the UP value.

Process Analytical Technology (PAT) is a conceptual approach to quality assurance calling for increased reliance on monitoring throughout a manufacturing (or other) process rather than dependence on a final-stage quarantine and testing approach. There are two elements of PAT relevant here: (1) the concept of frequent, functionally continuous monitoring of the process (the PATmon variable) and (2) the self-correcting, cybernetic nature of that monitoring (PATcyb), assuring that variable measurements out of specification (beyond the design space) will be automatically adjusted. The definitional model suggests that these two PAT variables are averaged to define a combined PAT value.

The three variables of combined PAT, Risk and Design Space (UP) are averaged in the beginning of the formula. These three variables are equal and equally important elements in the operational definition of QbD.

The final two elements of the model are intended simply to remind appliers that the quality levels achieved by the QbD approach are mitigated by variation from the Good Manufacturing Practices and from internal Standard Operating Procedures. These deltas negatively impact on compliance acceptance and on the product quality (and hence safety) that compliance is intended to assure.

Together the elements of this stochastic model provide (a) an operational definition that is intended to minimize the rope–wall–fan–snake arguments and (b) provide a common foundation for research and discussion about QbD. With a common understanding, pharmaceutical manufacturing companies can analyze the value of a QbD approach and begin experimenting with its implementation. FDA reviewers and investigators can provide consistent and effective guidelines for regulatory implementation. And, ultimately the public can be served with drugs and biologics that are safe, effective, and accessible.

4.4 QBD COST CONTAINMENT

Estimating the cost-containment contributions of QbD may be a bit problematic. Unlike most strategies discussed here, evolution to a QbD approach requires some affirmative investment before any cost savings can be realized.

While the Risk Assessment procedure is clearly cost-containing, and the Design Space, defining more flexible quality points, should lower costs, the increased monitoring and cybernetic controls of a Process Analytical Technology system may have some budgetary impact. Many organizations are already using PAT approach well in advance of the promulgation of QbD; but for those that have not adopted frequent and self-correcting monitoring equipment, additional software and hardware or the replacement of antiquated systems with more modern monitoring-inclusive equipment may be necessary.

It is difficult to determine the average amount of investment required, or the payback period to be expected. One manager of a major pharmaceutical company that implemented a QbD approach in a new manufacturing facility reported in confidence that the payback was under nine months: Almost immediately the cost savings of the new system surpassed the initial investment required. Those savings were a direct result of improved processing, reduced material waste, and reduced need to reprocess substandard material. The indirect costs of avoiding quarantine problems and resulting recalls would no doubt further accelerate the payback period.

Of course, should the FDA require (or even strongly encourage) a QbD approach to manufacturing, the cost-containment issue will quickly become moot. If QbD is state of the art for the industry and an expected and necessitated approach, the issue becomes one of minimizing the cost of QbD implementation rather than a comparison between the expense of having or not having a QbD system. In such a circumstance, likely to evolve over the next six to eight years, prior implementation of a PAT system will prove an effective cost-containment strategy: it is recommended that, beginning immediately, the key PAT monitoring elements should be included in any design proposal or request for proposal for any new or replacement manufacturing system component.

4.5 QbD IN LABORATORIES

Quality by Design (QbD) is an initiative of the US Food and Drug Administration and the biomedical industries it regulates and is intended to integrate the quality process through research, development, manufacturing, and distribution.[3] When properly implemented, QbD improves speed to market; reduces product variation; improves operating efficiency; and reduces costs at all stages of the process.

When applied to the automated laboratory, QbD principles provide continuous monitoring of all key variables, allowing scientists and managers to focus attention on the areas of the laboratory operation with the highest level of risk. In fact, the QbD approach integrates three key emerging regulatory concepts: Process Understanding, which identifies variable parameters and acceptable variances, focusing on **what** should be measured or monitored; Process Analytical Technology (PAT), which determines **how** those variables should be measured or monitored; and Risk Analysis, which establishes the **priority** of those measurements.

4.6 PROCESS UNDERSTANDING

In a laboratory setting, the process understanding step is generally included in the design of the laboratory, the selection of the laboratory equipment, and/or the design of the laboratory experiment. It is in those planning stages that critical decisions are made about the collection and processing of samples, the assays to be conducted, and the interpretative analyses to be applied to those assays.

These design space decisions are summarized in the study protocol and should include the decision criteria for acceptance or rejection (or re-analysis) of a test result. Appropriately, that decision criteria includes a range of acceptable and unacceptable result measurements.

While there is a wide range of laboratory testing models, most will include four steps:

Sample Manipulation and Control. Identification, plating, or other maneuver to mix sample with reagent and to enter sample into device; or to examine sample under varying magnification or manipulative conditions.

Testing and Data Measurement. The process of determining the reaction of the sample to the manipulation, and numerical characterization of that reaction.

---

[3] Snee, R. D., P. Cini, J. Kamm, and C. Meyers. Quality by Design—Shortening the Path to Acceptance, *Pharma Processing*, February 2008.

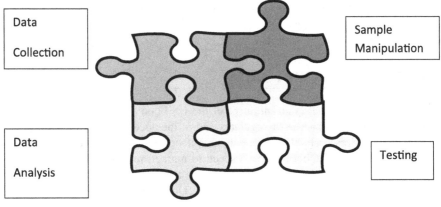

Figure 4.2

Data Collection. The reporting of those measurements to a database carefully tied to the sample identification.

Data Analysis. The statistical interpretation of the collected data to provide graphic, numerical, and or/label results.

When carefully and operationally defined, these four steps provide a composite picture of the design space, along with a clear delineation of the process or processes (Figure 4.2).

4.7 PROCESS ANALYTICAL CONTROL (PAT)

Process Analytical Control (PAT) has been recently endorsed by the FDA as a major component of manufacturing and analysis quality control.[4] Widely used in other industries (particularly chemical and petroleum), as well as used under a variety of different names in the pharmaceutical industry, PAT is a process of monitoring the performance of variables and functions identified in the Process Understanding procedures.

PAT has three basic components: two that are critical to the definition of process analytical control, and a third that represents a secondary implication with powerful value. A PAT system is characterized by continuous[5] measurements, by cybernetic responses to those measurements, and potentially by the capability of remote monitoring.

[4] Weinberg, S., Process Analytical Technology for Chromatography, *Journal of Chromatographic Sciences*, Vol. 44, March 2006.

[5] Actually, PAT measures are not continuous but are rapid multiple discrete measurements—but they are treated as though they are continuous in most analyses.

It is, of course, possible to (a) design a process without any quality checkpoints until the final stage and (b) presumably quarantine the end product of that process pending successful passing of a final stage test. The processing of human blood, for example, follows this model. A blood bag and two test tubes are collected (one tube is for testing, the other is for archive) and identified. After the processing of the bag, which takes only a few minutes, that bag of whole blood, plasma, cells, and so on, is refrigerated and stored awaiting the longer testing process. Meanwhile, and for several hours thereafter, the test tube of blood is examined for possible HIV, hepatitis, and other contaminations. When the tests are completed, the quarantined bag is retrieved and either labeled as safe for use or destroyed. While it is a necessary procedure in this instance, such a process is dangerous and inefficient: Quarantine errors, mislabeling, and other problems can have serious consequences.

In most circumstances there is a safer, higher-quality alternative. Under a PAT system, measurements of product purity and other characteristics can be collected at every stage of the process. The manufacture of penicillin, for example, requires the fermentation for several weeks of a mixture of grain, animal blood, water, and spores. Variations in temperature, pressure, or appropriate mixture agitation can kill the spores and prevent the growth of the penicillin. With continuous measurements, however, those variations can be quickly noted and corrected.

It is better to have an automated system like a thermostat or equivalent to self-correct the "out-of-spec" measurement than to have a human quality control professional note the variations on a gauge and thus making appropriate adjustments. The cybernetic process represents the second leg of the PAT procedure. In the penicillin fermentation chamber, for example, sensors can increase or decrease temperature, adjust the pressure, and turn on or off the agitator without awaiting the action of a quality control person. The result is much more rapid, more certain, and less subject to human error.

The final PAT characteristic is not fundamental to the concept, but may represent a secondary benefit. Because PAT in effect automates a part of the quality control process, the use of PAT permits remote monitoring of a laboratory or manufacturing system. Using the web or another connection, it is possible to centralize monitoring in a single station, with subsequent seamless human oversight and easy access by invited outside experts. With a remote monitoring system, an organization could consult with an expert on a particular problem; could permit temporary access by FDA regulators to discuss a strategy; and could lower monitoring costs with a centralized facility. The power industry has implemented this model: GE Energy has constructed a centralized monitoring station (located in a suburb of Atlanta, Georgia, USA) that monitors processes and safety at power plants around the world.[6]

While the remote capability does require some access control and security restrictions and may require special FDA-access policies, it does represent a valuable step in the QbD concept. With remote monitoring, continuous monitoring, and cybernetic controls, PAT presents the measurement of the key process points identified and supplies a critical piece of the QbD picture.

---

[6]Private tour, June 2006.

4.8   RISK ANALYSIS

The concept of risk analysis was first borrowed from the review process for medical devices in 2001 and was applied to 21 CFR Part11, the regulation of computer systems.[7] While Part 11 theoretically applied to all computer systems in use at a pharmaceutical organization, emphasis was clearly placed on the high-risk systems in which a control error would directly impact human health and safety.

In recent years the FDA has applied the risk analysis to all areas of regulation.[8] As the third critical element in QbD, the risk analysis allows prioritization of the quality measurements, guiding the process of determining which variables are most important and determining the degree of variance acceptable for each variable.

Once there is a clear understanding of the laboratory testing (or manufacturing, or development) process, along with a clear scheme for the measurement (using a PAT approach) of that process, the system manager is left with a dilemma. With a thorough identification of variables, along with near-constant measurement of those variables, there is a vast quantity of data containing minor variations in values. Is a 2% variance in the pill stamping pressure significant? Does a small spray variant on a capsule label painter have a real impact? Does at 0.005% evaporation on a liquid formulation adversely affect product strength?

To answer these kinds of questions and to focus on the important variations without drowning in the trivia or insignificant deviations, a risk assessment can provide defensible parameters and decision criteria. In the broadest terms, those variations that impact health and safety are important, whereas those that do not are generally considered insignificant.[9]

4.9   QbD IMPLICATIONS

The use of a QbD approach is not currently mandatory, and the concept in still evolving. The first trials of QbD submissions are currently underway, and most QbD attention has focused on the manufacturing process. Application of QbD to laboratory settings is just beginning to emerge, and formal guidelines and regulations are probably five to eight years away.

But the consideration of a QbD construct in planning, operating, and evaluating a laboratory operation has immediate value. In fact, it is likely that many laboratories will adopt QbD well in advance of any FDA mandate, yet another instance of the industry-driving new regulation.[10]

---

[7] Weinberg, S. The FDA Vector: Part 11 Risk-Based Changes, *American Biotechnology Laboratory*, May 2003.

[8] Weinberg, S. Regulation of Computer Systems, in *Computer Applications in Pharmaceutical Research and Development*, Chapter 26, Ekins, S., ed., John Wiley & Sons, Hoboken, NJ, 2006.

[9] Exception: Some minor variations, not directly affecting health and safety, serve as a "coal mine canary" warning of potential future impact on important variables.

[10] See, for example, Weinberg, S. Cost-Effective Compliance, *Scientific Computer and Instrumentation*, March 2003.

Regardless of the state of FDA acceptance or requirement, QbD provides a management framework with significant financial incentives to make it attractive. Quality problems detected post-application require product rejection (in a quarantine system) or recycling (in a fill line, for example). In a laboratory, post-analysis quality errors at best require a rerun of a test or experiment; at worst, the problem could corrupt results and lead to expensive erroneous conclusions.

With a QbD approach the laboratory process begins with a clear analysis of the test process: a step critical to system design, equipment selection, and experimental design. It next implements a continuous stream of quality checks, rapidly signaling significant variants from experimental design, equipment problems, operating failures, and process errors. Those problems may be cybernetically self-corrected, or may warn the laboratory operator to halt the process until a correction can be implemented.

Finally, a QbD approach provides a risk assessment that identifies the appropriate focus of the laboratory operations and provides a defensible justification for tolerances of variations. The effect may be (a) extended life of otherwise arbitrarily discarded reagents, (b) useful data from slightly contaminated samples, and (c) a more efficient laboratory operating procedure.

While a cost justification of a QbD approach must await more diverse industry experience with QbD implementation in laboratories, preliminary results for QbD in manufacturing suggest a rapid payback and a strong cost/benefit ratio.[11]

Quality by Design is a conceptualization rapidly gaining traction in the biomedical industries, led by an FDA initiative to reduce costs, increase quality control, and shift the primary responsibility for quality assurance firmly onto the industry. While initially focusing on the manufacturing sector, QbD is increasingly being adopted by automated laboratories. In that laboratory setting, where processes focus on sample control, testing, data collection, data analysis, and decision-making, Process Analytical Technology can provide continuous, cybernetic, and potentially centralized remote monitoring. At the same time, an effective Risk Analysis can define acceptable limits on parameters, prioritize those parameters, and assign appropriate foci on the most important and critical of the measured variables.

Over the next 10 years, QbD is likely to evolve into the dominate paradigm for biomedical quality. Current applications of QbD are rapidly infusing the manufacturing industry. As initial trials prove successful, QbD submissions are likely to dominate that sector over the next two to three years. Laboratories are adopting QbD procedures, with formal guidelines and regulations anticipated in approximately five to eight years. And the applications of QdB to clinical studies, already in exploratory stages, should reach critical levels within the decade.

The rationale behind the expected evolution to QbD dominance is based upon two critical factors. First, QbD is comprehensive: It incorporates all three aspects of quality control and assurance. QbD includes (a) an approach to identification and analysis of the processes underlying the system, (b) a methodology for measuring

[11] Nee, R. D., L. B. Hare, and J. R. Trout, *Experiments in Industry—Design, Analysis and Interpretation of Results*, Quality Press, Birmingham, AL, 1985.

and cybernetically controlling those processes, and (c) a risk-based prioritization and interpretation of those measurements.

Secondly, QbD is logically consistent. It provides a rational framework for controlling quality in production, search, laboratories, and other requirements, with a reasonable and defensible system of tolerances and permissible variants. QbD makes good sense for the management of an automated laboratory: Understand the processes involved, measure the performance of those processes, and interpret those measurements in a risk construct.

With reasonable assurance, a QbD approach to laboratory quality control and assurance will be the dominant paradigm of the future.

4.10 SUMMARY

Quality by Design (QbD) is an evolving initiative of the US Food and Drug Administration, simplified from more extensive and rigorous methodologies of the same name in use in the general manufacturing engineering industries. In its current configuration, QbD includes (a) the use of a Risk Assessment to determine which variables and parameters are most important in the quality control of a product, (b) the use of a Design Space analysis to determine the effective range or variance of those variables, and (c) the use of a Process Analytical Technology approach to continuously monitor and cyberneticly adjust those variables. Once implemented, QbD can greatly improve quality assurance and control while containing costs; the investment necessary to cd xposition a system for QbD varies widely. It is likely to represent a cost increase (with reasonable payback period) until regulatory guidelines and/or industry standards force that investment.

Quality by Design is therefore likely to represent a short-term cost increase but a long-term effective cost containment strategy, and it is likely to be a mandatory norm within the next two to five years.

CHAPTER 5

OUTSOURCING

5.1 INTRODUCTION

"Outsourcing" involves the use of subcontractors and/or consultants to fill specific staff roles. At one extreme is the virtual company, where a small cadre of executives outsource to a variety of Contract Research Organizations (CROs), Contract Manufacturing Organizations (CMOs), regulatory consultants, technical writers, and other freelancers to provide all or most of the functions of pharmaceutical, device, or biologics company. At the other extreme is the large established company that occasionally uses a highly specialized consultant for a short-duration, clearly defined task. Most organizations fall between these extremes, calling on professional organizations, individuals, and companies to assist with long- or short-term activities.

Although all of these outsourcing agencies are charging a premium to cover their own personnel, marketing, and management costs, the use of subcontractors and consultants can actually be a successful cost-containing strategy. Many organization use outsourcing largely to control headcount and to provide flexibility in the event of a downturn, but there are direct savings to be had even though a consultant generally costs 30% to 50% more than an equivalent full-time employee.

For global companies, the flexibility may be the driving force that leads to subcontractors, without consideration of possible savings. Within most European countries, for example, strict hiring laws may significantly restrict the ability of a company to lay off, reduce in force, or even reassign long-term employees. In such an environment the use of consultants permits an ongoing relationship without restricting work rules. In global companies operating in the United States and Europe, exclusive use of full-time employees can result in laying off of US workers even as possible less-qualified European workers (protected by local employment laws) are retained; using subcontractors can correct this imbalance.

But even without this secondary advantage and despite the premium charged by outside companies to cover their own costs of operations and profit, the use of subcontractors and consultants can prove an effective cost-containment strategy. The key issue in the savings to be realized lies in the expertise of those outsourcing agencies.

Cost-Contained Regulatory Compliance: For the Pharmaceutical, Biologics, and Medical Device Industries, First Edition. Sandy Weinberg.

5.2 THE VALUE OF EXPERTISE

The old joke that was previously stated in Chapter 3 about the building manager and the expert plumber applies here as well. The expert knows where to tap the boiler.

The problem with a good employee is that he or she must be a generalist in order to be effective. If the staff statistician, for example, has devoted her career to very detailed nonparametric analyses, she may not be productive when dealing with the daily variety of statistics questions that arise. A staff engineer must have a general knowledge of the entire manufacturing system; and effective regulatory professional should have an understanding of all the documents and processes the FDA requires. But that effective generalist may not be the ideal person to deal with the problems of a particular robotic sample transport system, or to cope with the intricacies of an orphan drug Investigatory New Drug Application. Unless the company submits orphan INDs on a regular basis, or is having continuous problems with the sample system, having a specialist on staff is an unnecessary and expensive luxury.

Of course in very large companies enough divisions may be working on orphans, or enough different sample systems may be used, to justify keeping on staff a specialist who serves as an "in-house consultant," loaned out throughout a vast global company on specific projects as needed. This pool of in-house specialists probably explains the rather limited use of outsourcing in large companies: The larger the organization, the more likelihood it can "in-source" rather than outsource. But the need for well-trained, experience specialists remains relatively constant.

There are two aspects of the expertise needed to solve emerging pharmaceutical, biologics, and device problems. First, to maximize cost containment, that expertise should include an element of experience. And second, to assure the credibility of the solutions devised, that expertise must be supported by appropriate credentials.

Experience is an effective teacher when accompanied by an analysis of what has worked (or not worked) and why. Remember that if a cat sits on a hot stove, it will quickly learn never to do so again; but the cat will never sit on a cool stove, either. When tempered by effective expert analysis, experience can be invaluable in providing models and solutions and in providing templates for future use. It is experience that can most effectively tell you "where to tap." A specialist may, over time, develop a rich experience in solving a specific category or problem that can quickly and cost effectively identify and implement solutions.

With effective training and education to back up that experience, the specialist not only can put experience into better perspective, analyzing the differing characteristics of a hot and cold stove, but also can bring credibility to the problem that is critical importance in a highly regulated environment. In the pharmaceutical, device, and biologics industries, it is not enough to be in control; you must also demonstrate that control to the FDA. A credentials expert can be the key to that demonstration.

With the training and education (and resulting credentials) to effectively analyze a variety of experiences, along with the pool of that experience to help identify problems and effectively implement solutions, the organization has the expertise to prevent or solve crises and has the credibility to demonstrate that expertise to regulatory authorities. In maintaining working production lines, reducing the likelihood of recalls, preventing negative regulatory findings and the resulting delays and adverse publicity, and minimizing the necessity of reprocessing or discarding substandard product, access to that expertise can clearly be a cost-containment strategy. And unless the organization is so large as to keep a pool of experts busy on a continuous basis, the most cost-effective method of obtaining that expertise is through outsourcing.

5.3   OUTSOURCE CRITERIA

If, as proposed, the major or primary value of outsourcing is the expertise and experience that can be applied to a problem or environment, it is clear that the major criteria in selecting subcontractors and consultants must be the credentials of the individuals to be utilized. Perhaps surprisingly, these are not the criteria most often utilized.

All too often, outsource individuals are selected on the basis of (a) the reputation of the umbrella organization supplying the "experts" or (b) the relationship of the company seeking assistance with that umbrella organization. Some major national (and international) consulting firms do not even supply actual proposed project participant resumes for review, providing instead "typical profiles" or generalized generic resumes. If the hiring organization does try to review resumes or interview proposed candidates, the vetting process is often left to human resource professionals without the specific knowledge and skills necessary to evaluate real expertise. The result may be a team of persons who closely resemble and replicate the in-house personnel they are supplementing. This approach may be successful for virtual organizations or for organizations seeking assistance without added permanent headcount, but is a less successful strategy if the goal is to bring in real focused expertise for a specific need. The cost containment that can be expected from finding the expert who "knows where to tap the boiler" requires a detailed and function evaluation of the proposed outsourcing candidates.

The criteria for that expertise fall into five general categories: regulatory qualification, situational experience, problem experience, problem credentials, and managerial expertise. Every outsourcing candidate expected to produce significant cost containment through intervention should qualify in all five areas, with the depth and breadth of that qualification varying by situation.

"Regulatory qualification" refers to recent (within three years) training in the Good Manufacturing Practices (cGMPs) or one of the appropriate subsets (Good Laboratory Practices, GLPs; Good Clinical Practices, GCP, etc.) These general regulatory guidelines provide the framework and philosophy of operating in an FDA-regulated environment; all employees in an organization, whether full time or outsourcing temporaries, should be so qualified. In a contract research organization (CRO), for example, all personnel involved in an outsourced project should be subject to an initial screening for GCP training, or GCP training should be mandated as a part of their project orientation. Any individual involved with the project who does not understand the content and philosophy of the GCPs (or other appropriate

GxP guidelines) potentially contaminates the project, leaving open suspicion of undocumented work, fraud, sloppy procedures, and so on.

An ideal outsourcing candidate has prior experience with the kind of company and kind of product involved. This situational experience lends a likelihood that proposed problem approaches will be appropriate and targeted. An individual whose career has been focused exclusively in medical devices may not be appropriate for a drug manufacturing environment even if both settings involve establishing computer driven assembly lines. The unique characteristics of batch processing and accounting for individual capsules may not automatically translate. While direct experiential match is not a mandatory criterion, the closer the situational experience, the more likely the consultant's expertise will apply. To a lesser degree, an understanding of and experience with the subcontracting (hiring) organization is a useful but not necessary criterion. Understanding the organization's mission, structure, and environment are valuable pluses, enhancing the situational experience.

Experience with the particular problem area or project requirements is perhaps the most important selection criterion. It is this prior exposure, complete with trials, errors, and eventual successes, that will produce the core of any savings to be realized. Hiring an outsourced consultant is an expensive proposition: The payback is a direct result of the time saved in having full-time staff analyze a problem, explore possible avenues, and eventually identify the most productive path. The successful consultant offsets that expense by dividing that learning and trial time among all present, past, and future clients. If the consultant is approaching a problem without relevant prior experience, the saving produced will be significantly reduced. While a genius or genuinely luck outsider may stumble across a solution without prior experience, the odds of success are much greater with a person who can say "Ah, yes, I've seen that problem before—and know the solution."

"Problem credentials" refer to the credibility of the outsider. While related, credentials and experience are not identical. But the credentials of the consultant— the degrees, pedigree, resume, publication history, and packaging—of that person will go far toward selling the solution to the full-time staff of the organization and to the regulatory authorities reviewing the results. While project, ideas, problem solutions, and approaches should be evaluated on their own merits, individuals lacking in detailed expertise are often forced to use the credibility of the recommender to distinguish a practical idea from an unworkable solution.

The final criterion is the most commonly neglected: managerial expertise. This does not refer to the ability to direct large groups, or the administer teams in accordance with the culture and demands of the base organization: those skills may be necessary on all or even most projects. But the fundamental principles of managerial leadership—the ability to focus on and define a problem, to analyze and evaluate possible solutions, and to communicate the selected solution to the employees who will be responsible for implementation—transcend all outsourcing situations. If the consultant can't communicate clearly to and from the people he/she is assigned to help, the project is likely to flounder and the costs are unlikely to be successful contained. Because the outsourced consultant or subcontractor is an adjunct to rather than an integrated member of the core team, this managerial expertise is of greater importance that it would be within the hiring company. As any experience consultant will confirm, the key to a successful project is client management.

When these five criteria are met, the outsourced consultant (or, in rare cases, the subcontracting team) will provide the cost-containment strategic advantage sought. Without these characteristics, a subcontractor may help with headcount management, with flexibility in hiring, and with rapid staff-up for short-term needs. But to result in lower or control costs, consultants should have regulatory qualification, situational experience, problem experience, problem credentials, and managerial expertise.

5.4 SUMMARY

Outsourcing can be an effective cost-containment regulatory strategy despite the override charges representing an outside consulting of subcontracting organization's management fees and profit. The savings accrue from the careful selection of specific professionals who can bring time- and expense-saving expertise and specific experience. Key to these savings is the careful selection of those professionals and the detailed vetting of selected individuals to be certain that they bring real expertise and directly applicable experience.

All too many organizations make the mistake of deferring the selection and vetting of consultants and subcontractors to outsourcing organizations. These organizations have a vested interest in presenting some candidate, regardless of qualification, for a project. They may find themselves pressured to stretch the degree of expertise of the direct applicability of experience of a candidate. And unless the outsider brings to the table expertise that is otherwise missing from the organization, and experience that can directly increase the efficiency of a project, the cost savings and containment will not be realized.

Outsourcing has a number of important advantages other than cost containment: coping with temporary overloads, adding short-term manpower where needed, allowing full-time staff to focus on special projects, and so forth. But the cost-containment advantages flow directly from their ability to complete a job more rapidly and more accurately than the organizational staff. Unless the subcontractors and consultants can bring these advantages home, they will not successfully contain regulatory costs.

APPENDIX TO CHAPTER 5

The Outsourcing text in this chapter is supplemented by a very important, though obscure, document: It is the only readily identified document in which the FDA attempts to define the credentials of potential "outsource" consultants. This document is frequently cited in Federal courts during *voir dire* discussions of the credentials of expert witnesses.

The following FDA document, **Independent Consultants for Biotechnology Clinical Trial Protocols**, provides definitions of qualifications for consultants utilized by biologics companies and includes a clear definition of "independence."

INDEPENDENT CONSULTANTS FOR BIOTECHNOLOGY CLINICAL TRIAL PROTOCOLS

Guidance for Industry: Independent Consultants for Biotechnology Clinical Trial Protocols

US Department of Health and Human Services
Food and Drug Administration
Center for Biologics Evaluation and Research (CBER)
Center for Drug Evaluation and Research (CDER)
August 2004

For questions on the content of this document, contact Leonard Wilson, CBER, at 301-827-0373 or Susan Johnson, CDER, at 301-594-3937.

Additional copies of this guidance are available from:

Office of Communication, Training, and
Manufacturers Assistance, HFM-40
Center for Biologics Evaluation and Research
Food and Drug Administration
Suite 200N
1401 Rockville Pike
Rockville, MD 20852
Internet: http://www.fda.gov/cber/guidelines.htm
Phone: 800-835-4709 or 301-827-1800

Cost-Contained Regulatory Compliance: For the Pharmaceutical, Biologics, and Medical Device Industries, First Edition. Sandy Weinberg.
© 2011 John Wiley & Sons, Inc. Published 2011 by John Wiley & Sons, Inc.

or

Office of Training and Communication
Division of Communications Management
Drug Information Branch, HFD-210
Center for Drug Evaluation and Research
Food and Drug Administration
5600 Fishers Lane
Rockville, MD 20857
Phone: 301-827-4573
Internet: http://www.fda.gov/cder/guidance/index.htm

TABLE OF CONTENTS

Guidance for Industry[1]:
Independent Consultants for Biotechnology Clinical Trial Protocols
Contains Nonbinding Recommendations

This guidance document represents the agency's current thinking on this topic. It does not create or confer any rights for or on any person and does not operate to bind FDA or the public. An alternative approach may be used if such approach satisfies the requirements of the applicable statutes and regulations. If you want to discuss an alternative approach, contact the appropriate FDA staff. If you cannot identify the appropriate FDA staff, call the appropriate number listed on the title page of this guidance.

I. WHY IS FDA ISSUING THIS GUIDANCE?

On June 12, 2002, the President signed the Public Health Security and Bioterrorism Preparedness and Response Act of 2002, which included the Prescription Drug User Fee Amendments of 2002 (PDUFA III). Secretary Thompson's letter to Congress concerning PDUFA III included an addendum containing the performance goals and programs intended to facilitate the development and review of human drugs to which the Food and Drug Administration (FDA) had committed. The letter and addendum can be found on the Internet at http://www.fda.gov/oc/pdufa/default.htm.

---

[1] This guidance has been prepared by the Center for Biologics Evaluation and Research (CBER) and the Center for Drug Evaluation and Research (CDER) at the Food and Drug Administration.

One commitment was the establishment of a program that allows you, a sponsor of clinical trials for certain products, to request that we, FDA, engage an independent consultant to participate in the review of your protocol for a clinical study that is intended to serve as the primary basis of a claim of efficacy. We are publishing this guidance to explain when and how you may take advantage of this program. This guidance finalizes the draft guidance of the same title dated May 2003.

FDA's guidance documents, including this guidance, do not establish legally enforceable responsibilities. Instead, guidances describe FDA's current thinking on a topic and should be viewed only as recommendations, unless specific regulatory or statutory requirements are cited. The use of the word "should" in FDA's guidances means that something is suggested or recommended, but not required.

II. WHAT PRODUCTS ARE ELIGIBLE FOR THIS PROGRAM?

This program is available for a subset of products covered by PDUFA III. Your product qualifies for this program if:

- It is biotechnology-derived (for example, DNA plasmid products, synthetic peptides of fewer than 40 amino acids, monoclonal antibodies for *in vivo* use, and recombinant DNA-derived products),
- It has the potential to represent a significant advance in the treatment, diagnosis, or prevention of a disease or condition, or to address an unmet medical need, and
- The clinical study at issue is intended to serve as the primary basis of a claim of efficacy.

III. HOW DO YOU REQUEST THAT FDA ENGAGE AN INDEPENDENT CONSULTANT?

We recommend that you submit a written request to us asking that we engage a consultant as part of your request for a formal meeting, (e.g., an End of Phase 2 meeting.) You should clearly designate this as a "Request for Appointment of Expert Consultant." The request should include the information needed for the meeting as explained in FDA's "Guidance for Industry: Formal Meetings with Sponsors and Applicants for PDUFA Products,"[2] dated February 2000, and the reasons that you believe an expert consultant should be engaged. These reasons might include preliminary discussions with FDA that resulted in disagreement over the protocol or a novel or unorthodox approach to the clinical trial or its analysis.

IV. DOES YOUR REQUEST AFFECT THE PDUFA MEETING MANAGEMENT GOALS?

Yes. We will need time to select and screen the consultant for potential conflicts of interest and the consultant will need sufficient time to review the scientific issues involved. Therefore, we will extend certain of the performance goals for scheduling and holding a

[2] See www.fda.gov/cber/guidelines.htm

meeting by 60 days. We will notify you within 14 days of our intent to schedule your meeting and engage an independent consultant. We will not be able to tell you when the meeting will be scheduled until we have engaged the consultant. Similarly, if you wish the independent consultant to participate in other protocol assessment activities, such as a special protocol assessment and agreement, we will extend PDUFA performance goals related to those activities by sixty (60) days, to take into account the time necessary to select and screen the consultant. The goal for any given meeting management activity will be extended by not more than 60 days. It is our intention to schedule these activities as efficiently as possible.

V. HOW MANY TIMES CAN YOU USE THIS PROGRAM DURING THE DEVELOPMENT OF YOUR PRODUCT?

We will engage an independent consultant under this program only once during the development of your product. This restriction does not limit your ability to request that we take to an Advisory Committee an issue pertaining to the product's marketing application review. Nor does it limit our ability to take an issue to an Advisory Committee or otherwise to seek advice on an issue.

VI. CAN YOU RECOMMEND CONSULTANTS FOR THE FDA TO ENGAGE?

You can submit a list of recommended consultants, their qualifications, and contact information for us to consider. Prospective consultants will be screened for conflicts of interest. We suggest that you do not recommend consultants:

- Whom you know to have financial conflicts,
- Who have been involved in the design or planning of the clinical trial, or
- Whom you intend to ask to be an investigator.

We may or may not select the consultant from your list of recommendations. We will notify you of our selection prior to the formal meeting.

VII. WHAT IS THE STATUS AND ROLE OF THE CONSULTANT?

Prospective consultants will be screened for potential conflicts of interest according to the criteria described in Policies and Procedures for Handling Conflicts of Interest with FDA Advisory Committee Members, Consultants, and Experts[3] (FDA Waiver Criteria 2000) and be subject to confidentiality requirements. The consultant we select may or may not already be a special government employee. The consultant may:

- Review the clinical protocol and appropriate background material,
- Participate in our meeting with you, and
- Provide us with advice on your clinical protocol and product development plan.

We will remain responsible for making scientific and regulatory decisions regarding the clinical protocol, taking into account the consultant's advice.

Following the completion of their service with respect to this program, consultants that we retain under contract are not restricted from other interactions with FDA. These consultants will continue to be subject to the restrictions applicable to that position.[3]

VIII.   WILL WE ALWAYS GRANT YOUR REQUEST?

We will grant your request unless we determine that engaging an expert consultant would not serve a useful purpose (e.g., it is clearly premature).

- If we grant your request: We will engage an independent consultant, of our choosing.
- If we deny your request: We will provide you with a written rationale for the denial within 14 days of receipt of your request for an expert consultant.
- If you disagree with our rationale for refusing the request: You may submit a request for formal dispute resolution.

[3] See http://www.fda.gov/oc/advisory/conflictofinterest/intro.html

CHAPTER 6

ELECTRONIC SUBMISSIONS

6.1 INTRODUCTION

One strategy for maximizing cost containment is to focus on the most significant cost factors. If you are running an airline and your greatest controllable cost is fuel, it is there you focus your attention. If you are an international fast food franchise, perhaps advertising costs represent your greatest expenditure; and methods of minimizing ad expense by piggybacking with soft drink manufacturers, for example, becomes a priority. Rarely are significant savings realized by looking for pennies in the small expenditures; examining the big ticket items and seeking reduction strategies is generally a better tactic. Perhaps surprisingly, the greatest cost in the pharmaceutical, biologics, and device industries is directly related to time.

A US Patent provides protection (in exchange for disclosure) for a period currently set at 20 years. Unlike some countries in which that 20-year period begins with approval of a product, the US Freedom of Information Act makes the submission of a New Drug Application (NDA), Biologics License Application (BLA), or Medical Device Application a public disclosure, requiring the filing of the patent prior to regulatory submission.

Incidentally, this difference in patent law effect between the United States and most other nations accounts for a significant portion of the disparity in drug prices To determine the research and development chargeback for a drug developed in Belgium, for example, divide the development price by 20 (for the 20 years of the patent period). For the same drug in the United States, where the approval process can easily eat up eight or more years of the patent, divide the development costs by 12. The end result in drug price is significant.

As the FDA reviews, questions, awaits answers, ponders, and eventually (hopefully) approves the application, the patent clock is running, losing the time for exclusive marketing of the product and hastening the day when a generic equivalent can drive down price and capture market share. In the medical device area the effect may not be significant: Most devices are accepted (or rejected) within six months. But it is not unusual for an NDA or BLA to drag on for years, costing the company an estimated $25 million per day in lost revenue.[1]

---

[1] O'Mera, Alex. *Chasing Medical Miracles*, Walker Publishing, Reno, NV, 2009.

Cost-Contained Regulatory Compliance: For the Pharmaceutical, Biologics, and Medical Device Industries, First Edition. Sandy Weinberg.
© 2011 John Wiley & Sons, Inc. Published 2011 by John Wiley & Sons, Inc.

Any tool or technique that can shorten the review time represents significant cost containment. And to date, the most effective way of speeding the preparation, review, modification, and eventual approval of a new drug or biologic product is the use of electronic submissions.

The time gained falls into two categories: (a) increased speed and efficiency on the part of the submitting company and (b) increased speed and efficiency on the part of the US Food and Drug Administration. Unfortunately, the savings at the FDA end have not been as dramatic as the potential, though this is improving. Increased speed of submission and response by submitting companies has represented significant cost containment and is likely to generate even greater savings in the future.

An investigatory new drug application (IND) can easily run 10 or more volumes, largely consisting of reviews and copies of published studies of the drug in questions. An NDA or BLA may consist of thousands of pages of clinical data in addition to the documents detailing (a) the design of those studies and (b) directions for researchers conducting the studies (the Investigators' Brochure). Assembling, transmitting, and managing that volume of materials is a major task in itself, particularly if paper copies are used.[2] And again, each day used to check to make certain that all copies have complete versions with every page included and numbered represent significant lost revenue as the patent continues to run.

Most applications result in some follow up questions from the FDA. These questions may necessitate insertion of additional materials in the NDA or BLA; corrections; or other changes. Readjusting the page numbers for the table of contents can be a formidable task; if the changes can not be handled with an addendum, a new paper copy may need to be reprinted, reproofed, and resubmitted. Again, without an electronic submission, valuable days may be lost.

Many companies use a further cost-containment strategy of simultaneous submission to both FDA and EMEA.[3] Reformatting and modifications are obviously much more simple with an electronic submission, and again modifications can be handled much more efficiently.

An electronic submission can also significantly ease—and speed—the burden on FDA reviewers. With hyperlinking the cross-checking of a cited reference with the actual article is a simple click process. Electronic indexing and searching can all but instantly find whether and where a specific issue is addressed. And the management of the multiple volumes of a complex application is simplified when that entire text is contained on one or two disks. In discussion of questions with submitting companies, the ability to get everyone literally on the same page and to move efficiently from the section in question to a specified response document can avoid delaying misunderstandings and confusion. And the mundane act of checking logistics, including complete page numbering, document inclusion, form completion, and other administrative matters, can be reduced from days to minutes.

With all of these advantages, it may be surprising that the FDA was so slow in accepting electronic submissions, and perhaps even more surprising is that the

---

[2] See Weinberg, S. *Guidebook to Drug Regulatory Submissions*, John Wiley & Sons, Hoboken, NJ, 2009.
[3] See Chapter 7.

agency often seems to prefer paper over electronic copies even today. In the early 1980s the author was a member of an industry–FDA panel attempting (obviously without success) to establish standards for electronic data management. Even by FDA standards, 20 + years is an unusually glacial pace. The reasons for the slow transition are complex, but finally standards of formatting and transmission are emerging. As test projects are completed, support organizations fine-tune their tools, and FDA personnel become familiar with common products, a series of de facto or de jure electronic submissions standards are likely to supplement the guidelines currently in place, and the use of electronic submissions will become the norm in the drug, biologics, and device industries—a major cost-containment development.

6.2   SECONDARY BENEFITS

The electronic submission of clinical and preclinical data provides a potential secondary benefit for both the industry as a whole and for individual submitting companies. This secondary benefit can provide substantial cost savings for the entire clinical testing process.

In addition to providing electronic text that is easily indexed and electronic citations that can be effectively hyperlinked, the submission includes what are in effect two electronic databases of clinical findings. The first database can be mined to find the significant and subtle effects of the drug, biologic, or device under investigation. Sophisticated statistical analyses can determine interactive effects, secondary side effects, counterindications with linked diseases, and other results of the protocol. The second database, consisting of control cases to whom the drug, device, or biologic was not administered, is used to isolate and identify placebo effects.

As the second "control" database grows over time, it can serve two important cost-containing functions. First, by matching subjects in the control database with subjects in a given experimental database, it may be possible to avoid the need for as many control patients in future clinical studies. In effect, the same patient might serve as a control in multiple experiments. Not only would this redundancy save some of the costs in clinical studies, but it would also eliminate a major ethical hurdle in clinical research: the withholding of treatment from a randomly selected control group to measure the true effects of a new therapy.

Second, as the control group database grows, it will be increasingly likely to provide information about the interactive effects of linked and of independent diseases. For example, it may be possible to study either (a) the effects of progressive heart disease on patients who are being actively treated for Type 2 Diabetes or (b) the effect on dementia with Lewy Body disease on patients undergoing treatment for Parkinson's disease. These findings would not only have potentially valuable research results, but could significantly contain the costs associated for clinical research in these areas.

These secondary benefits from electronic submissions (and from the commonly and cooperatively available databases the submissions produce) will not only help contain the costs of regulatory compliance but ought to have a significant impact on the costs—and time—involved in clinical trials. With the potential for overlapping control groups, we should reduce or eliminate the time required for recruiting clinical subjects, administering placebo therapies to the randomly selected (and blinded) control subjects, and following those individuals. And, again, time is money because patent protection is finite and fleeting.

6.3   SUBMISSION GUIDELINES

Electronic submissions are carefully reviewed in a three-step process. In step one, an administrator reviews the application to assure complete conformity to all appropriate guidelines and published Frequently Asked Questions (FAQs). This review will include all technical requirements for the submission (see FDA DOCUMENT in the appendix to this chapter), logistical requirements, pagination, and so on. Until all of these requirements have been met, the application is not reviewed by anyone with a content expertise.

In step two the submission is assigned to a reviewer, who examines the content for the first time. This review may take weeks or months, depending on the time and size of the submission. The review will examine and often replicate statistical analyses, will read many of the cited publications, and will examine the detailed technical specifications included in the submission. This second step generally concludes with a summary review and recommendation.

The recommendation of step two is then forwarded to a committee of FDA experts and/or outside experts, depending on the type of submission. This third step generally takes several weeks. The committee will rely heavily on the summary review and recommendation of the assigned reviewer, but may also examine the primary data and documents of the submission and may accept, reject, or modify the recommendation.

Table 6.1 shows a generalized electronic submission checklist.

6.4   BARRIERS TO STANDARDIZED ELECTRONIC SUBMISSION GUIDELINES

The development of formats and guidelines for electronic submissions has been a lengthy process and is still evolving. While a part of this process is a normal result of the cautious rate of progress in the agency, there are three specific barriers that are slowing the development of universal or common submission standards: diverse agency needs, industry difficulty in reaching agreement, and the relative speed of technological versus regulatory innovation.

Because the process of developing electronic submission guidelines has been more evolutionary than planned, each division within FDA has distinct and subtly different requirements. Drug, Biologics, Food, Veterinary, Device, and other FDA subgroups have established their own distinct sets of procedures, making it difficult for a third-party submission consulting group of software organization to

TABLE 6.1   Electronic Submission Checklist

☐ Form 1571 completed
☐ Cover letter
  ☐ Name and address of sponsor
  ☐ Name and address, title, telephone, e-mail of contact person
  ☐ Generic and trade name of drug or drug product or device
  ☐ FDA Code Number (assigned at time of pre-conference)
☐ Letter includes summary of action to date; planned action; and summary of any adverse
  events or outcomes.
☐ For NDAs/ANDAs: Updated CMC Information provided, including evidence of purity,
  stability, toxicology testing, and integrity of API, placebo, and final product.
☐ For NDA/ANDs: Drug Master File updated, including information on facilities, processes, and
  articles used in manufacturing, processing, packaging, and storage.
☐ For NDA/ANDAs: Investigators Brochure updated for all applicant conducted studies
  included with detailed information for investigators and IRB records.
☐ For NDA/ANDAs: Updated complete pharmacological profile provided for API and final
  product.
☐ Summary of adverse reactions to proposed drug.

---

effectively service the industry. Except for the largest of the drug development companies, those third-party organizations are critical managers of the submissions process, yet they tend not to specialize in one specific submissions target but rather to offer diverse services across the industry. This diversity of standards within the agency, coupled with the mismatch between submissions consulting firm business models and the needs of the industry, has slowed the electronic submissions process.

When different electronic formats are introduced in a marketplace—beta versus VCR, blue ray versus a variety of competitors, or Microsoft versus Apple—there are two possible outcomes: Either one competitor captures the market and forces out the other (as with VCRs); or the smaller of the two retreats to a stable niche market, as with Apple. But the convenience of having a near-universal standard quickly leads to an overwhelming dominance of a single mainstream format. Until a player achieves dominance, however, the market may languish in chaos seeking a standard; arguably, this is the fundamental reason for the cost differential between US and European cell phone rates.

Currently the FDA electronic submission field is still locked in the early competitive stage, awaiting the emergence of a dominant player. Recent developments with eCTD and SUGI26 suggest that the field will clear very rapidly over the next few years, with a coalition standard (probably led by SAS Institute) achieving standard acceptance. In the meantime the FDA will probably accept a variety of formats with a resulting delay from the learning curve and the training of FDA personnel in the use of particular format employed.

But there is a fundamental problem underlying that eventual definition of a standard electronic submissions format. Once adopted and institutionalized, it will be difficult to modify that format even as technological advances offer significant improvements and valued features. Given the speed of innovation in the computer field, along with the glacial rate of development of new guidelines at FDA—generally a process involving the formation of a committee, months of meetings to agree on wording, and a six-month or longer public comment period, followed by a revision prior to final release—any new standard is likely to be obsolete by the time it is promulgated. The FDA's standard for validation and control of computer systems (21 CFR Part 11) took more than four years of development, and then it was only useful because it established general principles rather than specific testing requirements.

This problem is likely to be solved in part through the adoption of standardized format system with a controlling panel or group that can update regularly, in effect bypassing normal FDA guideline release procedures. But given the need to familiarize FDA personnel with format changes and new features, the problems are likely to continue and to cost some of the efficiencies.

Despite these changes, electronic submissions represent a significant cost-containment strategy and are likely to be mandated by innovation pressures in advance of regulatory force.

6.5 SUMMARY

As current experiments in the use of and standards for utilization of electronic submissions continue to progress, a newly computerized Food and Drug Administration will emerge. With this modernization to accept submissions, analyze results, and cross-compare findings will come significant cost-containment regulatory opportunities.

Initially the widespread use of electronic submission of clinical trial-based NDA, BLA, and PMAs will reduce the review bottleneck and speed the review process, resulting in significant reduction of time lost while patent exclusivity is running. Over time, increased regulatory familiarity with the databases constituting those submissions will lead to cost savings in study designs as control groups are combined and interactive effects are modeled.

A more computerized, modernized, and automated FDA will likely lead to other cost-containment opportunities for the drug, device, and biologics industries as increased agency efficiency and improved industry-agency interaction permit more rapid, exact, and efficient regulatory compliance.

APPENDIX TO CHAPTER 6

Specific details on electronic submissions are now available for most regulatory submissions, but experience suggests that a review of FDA requirements and preferences might be an appropriate addition to the Pre-Submission meeting to assure that a specific team hasn't made any changes. At least as a starting point, the key guidance document is appended.

ELECTRONIC SUBMISSIONS, THE 2005 DOCUMENT THAT APPLIES TO CDER (PHARMACEUTICALS) AND CBER (BIOLOGICS) SUBMISSIONS

US Department of Health and Human Services
Food and Drug Administration
Center for Drug Evaluation and Research (CDER)
Center for Biologics Evaluation and Research (CBER)
October 2005

Additional copies are available from:

Division of Drug Information, HFD-240
Center for Drug Evaluation and Research
Food and Drug Administration
5600 Fishers Lane
Rockville, MD 20857
(Tel) 301-827-4573
http://www.fda.gov/cder/guidance/index.htm

and/or

Office of Communication, Training and
Manufacturers Assistance, HFM-40
Center for Biologics Evaluation and Research
Food and Drug Administration
1401 Rockville Pike
Rockville, MD 20852
http://www.fda.gov/cber/guidelines.htm

Cost-Contained Regulatory Compliance: For the Pharmaceutical, Biologics, and Medical Device Industries, First Edition. Sandy Weinberg.
© 2011 John Wiley & Sons, Inc. Published 2011 by John Wiley & Sons, Inc.

TABLE OF CONTENTS

    4. *Datasets*

    5. *Periodic Safety Update Reports*

    6. *Literature References*

IV. Utility Folder

    A. Document-Type Definition Folder

    B. Style Folder

Technical specifications associated with this guidance will be provided as stand-alone documents. They will be updated periodically. To ensure that you have the most recent versions, check the appropriate center's guidance Web page. For CBER, this Web site is http://www.fda.gov/cber/esub/esub.htm. For CDER, this Web site is http://www.fda.gov/cder/regulatory/ersr/ectd.htm.

Guidance for Industry[1]:

Providing Regulatory Submissions in Electronic Format—Human Pharmaceutical Product Applications and Related Submissions Using the eCTD Specifications

This guidance represents the Food and Drug Administration's (FDA's) current thinking on this topic. It does not create or confer any rights for or on any person and does not operate to bind FDA or the public. An alternative approach may be used if such approach satisfies the requirements of the applicable statutes and regulations. If you want to discuss an alternative approach, contact the FDA staff responsible for implementing this guidance. If you cannot identify the appropriate FDA staff, call the appropriate number listed on the title page of this guidance.

I. INTRODUCTION

This is one in a series of guidance documents intended to assist applicants making regulatory submissions to the FDA in electronic format using the electronic common technical document (eCTD) specifications. This guidance discusses issues related to the electronic submission of applications for human pharmaceutical products[2] and related submissions, including abbreviated new drug applications (ANDAs), biologics license applications (BLAs), investigational new drug applications (INDs), new drug application (NDAs), master files (e.g., drug master files), advertising material, and promotional labeling.[3] At this time, this does not include applications supporting combination products.

[1] This guidance has been developed by the Center for Drug Evaluation and Research (CDER) and the Center for Biologics Evaluation and Research (CBER).

[2] Human pharmaceutical products include those products that meet the definition of *drug* under the Food, Drug and Cosmetic Act, including those that are chemically synthesized and those derived from living sources (biologic products).

[3] Agency guidance documents on electronic submissions will be updated regularly to reflect the evolving nature of the technology and the experience of those using this technology.

Paperwork Reduction Act of 1995: This guidance contains information collection provisions that are subject to review by the Office of Management and Budget (OMB) under the Paperwork Reduction Act of 1995 (44 U.S.C. 3501-3520). The collections of information in this guidance have been approved under OMB Control Nos. 0910-0014, 0910-0001, and 0910-0338.

The goals of the guidance are to enhance the receipt, processing, and review of electronic submissions to the FDA. Specifically, this guidance makes recommendations regarding the use of the *eCTD backbone files* developed through the International Conference on Harmonisation (ICH) to facilitate efficient submission handling. In addition, the guidance provides more specificity than in previous guidances for electronic submissions with regard to the organization of individual submissions. Finally, the guidance harmonizes the organization and formatting of electronic submissions for multiple submission types.

This guidance refers to a series of technical specifications associated with the guidance. They are being provided as stand-alone documents to make them more accessible to the user. The associated specifications will be updated periodically. To ensure that you have the most recent versions, check the appropriate center's guidance Web page.

FDA's guidance documents, including this guidance, do not establish legally enforceable responsibilities. Instead, guidances describe the Agency's current thinking on a topic and should be viewed only as recommendations, unless specific regulatory or statutory requirements are cited. The use of the word *should* in Agency guidances means that something is suggested or recommended, but not required.

II. GENERAL ISSUES

This portion of the guidance makes recommendations on general organizational issues related to the electronic submission of applications for human pharmaceutical products using the cCTD specifications. The requirements for *the content* of such applications are described in our regulations in Chapter 21 of the Code of Federal Regulations (CFR). Additional recommendations on the contents of applications are provided in Agency guidances, which are available on the Agency Web page.

A. Scope

This guidance applies to marketing applications (ANDAs, BLAs, NDAs), investigational applications (INDs), and related submissions (master files, advertising material, and promotional labeling). The guidance applies equally to original submissions, supplements, annual reports, and amendments to these applications and related submissions, including correspondence. This guidance does not apply to electronic submission of prelicense or preapproval inspection materials.

B. Guidance on the Content of Applications and Related Submissions

This document provides general guidance on how to organize application information for electronic submission to the Agency using the eCTD specifications. Guidance on the information to be included in the technical sections of applications and submissions is described in a series of guidance documents based on the International Conference on Harmonisation of Technical Requirements for Registration of Pharmaceuticals for Human Use (ICH) common technical document (CTD): *M4: Organization of the CTD, M4Q: The CTD—Quality; M4S—The CTD Safety*; and *M4E: The CTD—Efficacy.*

C. ICH eCTD Specification

The recommendations made here on how to organize application information are based on the ICH CTD and the electronic CTD (eCTD), which was developed by the ICH M2 expert working group. Although the CTD and the eCTD were designed for marketing applications, they could apply equally to other submission types, including INDs, master files, advertising material, and promotional labeling.[4] Details on the specification for the ICH eCTD can be found in the guidance document *M2 eCTD: Electronic Common Technical Document Specification.*

D. Document Granularity and Table of Contents Headings

Submissions are a collection of documents. A document is a collection of information that includes forms, reports, and datasets. When making an electronic submission, *each document should be provided as a separate file.*[5] The documents, whether for a marketing application, an investigational application, or a related submission, should be organized based on the five modules in the CTD: module 1 includes administrative information and prescribing information, module 2 includes CTD summary documents, module 3 includes information on quality, module 4 includes the nonclinical study reports, and module 5 includes the clinical study reports.

A table of contents is defined by headings arranged in a hierarchical fashion. See the associated specification, Comprehensive Table of Contents Headings and Hierarchy for the comprehensive listing of headings and hierarchy. Because this is a comprehensive listing, not all headings are applicable to all submissions or submission types. All of the information you need to submit is covered by these headings. If you think other headings are needed, you should contact our electronic submission coordinators prior to using any other headings (see Section II.S of this guidance). Reviewers will not be able to access documents associated with headings not listed in the "Comprehensive Table of Contents Headings and Hierarchy."

Unless otherwise specified, documents should be organized so that the subject matter of the document is specifically associated with the lowest heading in the table of contents hierarchy. For example, if you look at the associated document "Comprehensive Table of Contents Headings and Hierarchy," the headings "Meeting request" and "Meeting background material" are the lowest headings in the "Meeting" hierarchy. Therefore, the meeting request and meeting background material would be in two separate documents— the meeting request in one document and the meeting background material in another document.

A document can be associated with more than one heading. However, the actual electronic file would only be provided once. The eCTD specifications provide details on how to refer to an electronic file.

E. Electronic Submissions

Under our regulations (21 CFR 11.2(b)(2)), applicants and sponsors are expected to contact us for details on how to proceed with electronic submissions. These details are usually provided in guidance documents. For example, we are already receiving marketing application submissions for human pharmaceutical products in electronic format based on details provided in the guidances for industry *Providing Regulatory Submissions in Electronic Format—NDAs, Providing Regulatory Submissions in Electronic Format— ANDAs, Providing Regulatory Submissions to the Center for Biologics Evaluation and*

---

[4] Advertising and promotional labeling provided with marketing applications.

[5] Some documents are provided in more than one file because a file containing everything would be too large. See specifications for the size limitations for a file.

Research (CBER) in Electronic Format—Biologics Marketing Applications, and *Providing Regulatory Submissions in Electronic Format—General Considerations.*[6] However, we recommend that you begin submitting eCTD backbone files as described in this guidance because we believe that having the information in the eCTD backbone files will result in greater efficiency in the future. In time, the other guidances may be withdrawn because they may no longer be needed.

When we are ready to receive a particular submission type in electronic format only, we usually identify it in public docket 92S-0251. Under 21 CFR part 11, you then have the option of providing that submission type in electronic format according to FDA guidance so that the Agency may adequately process, archive, and review the files.

Once you begin to submit a specific application in electronic format based on this guidance, subsequent submissions to the application, including amendments and supplements, should include eCTD backbone files. Without the eCTD backbone files, we will not be able to adequately manage, process, archive, or review the submissions. If you choose to submit an original application using the eCTD backbone files, you should obtain an application number in advance by contacting the appropriate center. You may obtain the number at any time and the numbers will not be reused.

We believe it is most beneficial to begin your eCTD-based submissions with the initial submission of an application. Contact the appropriate center first if you wish to make eCTD-based submissions to pending applications. You should avoid the submission of any paper documents when you follow the recommendations in this document. The maximum benefit will be derived once an application is in electronic format. This is particularly true for the IND, where submissions are provided over a long period of time. You should submit the electronic information for all files in the eCTD backbone files following the specifications associated with this guidance.

F.   Document Information for Previous Submissions

If you decide to submit a specific application in electronic format based on this guidance, you do not have to provide eCTD backbone files for the previous submissions to the application. For example, if you submitted an original application in 2001 and now submit an amendment to the application using the eCTD backbone files, you do not have to go back and submit the document information for the files submitted in 2001.

G.   Referencing Previously Submitted Documents[7]

If a document was submitted in electronic format with the eCTD backbone files, you should not submit additional copies when referencing the previously submitted document. Instead, you should include the information by reference by providing in the text of the document (1) the application or master file number, (2) the date of submission (e.g., letter date), (3) the document name, and (4) the page number of the referenced document along with a hypertext link to the location of the information (see Section II.Q of this guidance). If a document replaces or appends a document previously submitted with an eCTD back-

---

[6] This includes mixed electronic and paper submissions.

[7] Previously submitted documents include previously submitted information by reference for master files, market applications, and investigational applications discussed under 21 CFR 312.23(a)(11)(b), 314.50(g)(1), 314.420(b), and 601.51(a).

bone file, then you should include this information in the appropriate eCTD backbone file. The details on how to include this information in the eCTD backbone file are provided in the associated specifications for eCTD backbone files.

If a document was previously submitted in either paper or electronic format without the proper eCTD backbone files, you should reference the document as with any paper submission. In the text of the document, you should include (1) the application or master file number, (2) the date of submission (e.g., letter date), (3) the document name, (4) the page number, and (5) the submission identification (e.g., submission serial number, volume number, electronic folder, and file name) of the referenced document. In such cases, providing an electronic copy of the previously submitted documents can increase the utility of the submission. These documents, like all documents in the submission, should be appropriately described in the eCTD backbone files. These files are considered *new* in the eCTD backbone files.

When referring to documents that are part of other applications, please remember to include the appropriate letters of authorization with the submission (e.g., 21 CFR 314.420(d)).

H. Refuse to File

We may refuse to file an application or supplement under our regulations (e.g., 21 CFR 314.101 and 601.2) if the submission is illegible, uninterpretable, or otherwise clearly inadequate, including having incompatible formats or inadequate organization. These regulations apply to both paper and electronic submissions. The absence of electronic datasets in an acceptable format to permit review and analysis may be considered inadequate, resulting in a refuse-to-file decision.[8] Following the recommendations in this guidance document will help ensure that your electronic application meets the requirements of FDA regulations and can be archived, processed, and reviewed within specified time frames using our tools.

I. Submission of Paper Copies

When providing applications in electronic format using the eCTD backbone files, paper copies of the application, including review copies and desk copies, are not required and should not be sent.

J. Scanned Documents

Scanned documents submitted electronically as images are not as useful for review as documents that are text based. Image-based documents are more difficult to read and cannot be electronically searched. It takes longer to print image-based documents, and they occupy more storage space than text-based documents. For these reasons, we strongly urge that you provide text-based documents, rather than image files, whenever possible. We understand that certain documents may only be available as image files. Handwritten documents and documents that were generated independent from the company, such as journal publications, may be available only in paper. Documents that may only be available in paper can be scanned and submitted in electronic format as image-based files. However, we expect documents such as study reports recently generated by the company or recently

---

[8] See more on this in CBER's SOPP 8404.

generated as the result of the company's request to be available as text-based documents. We understand that legacy study reports, those generated years ago, may only be available in paper. For these reports, especially those for pivotal studies, you may want to consider converting these documents from image files to text-based files. Optical Character Recognition that has been validated is an option.

K. The FDA District Office Copy

FDA District offices have access to documents submitted in electronic format. Therefore, when sending submissions in electronic format, you need not provide any documentation to the FDA Office of Regulatory Affairs District Office.

L. Electronic Signatures

Documents required by regulations to be submitted with an original signature (e.g., FDA form 356h, FDA form 1571) should be submitted with electronic signatures that follow the controls described under 21 CFR part 11.

M. Number of Copies of Electronic Files

You should send a single copy of the electronic portions of a submission to the appropriate central document room facility. Copies should not be sent directly to the reviewer or review division. Electronic documents that bypass the controls for electronic files described in 21 CFR 11 are not considered official documents for review.

N. Naming Electronic Files

To function properly, the eCTD backbone files must have specific names (e.g., index.xml, us-regional.xml). For other files without a specified name, you should provide a name that is indicative of the contents (e.g., protocol-101). The file name should allow a reviewer to infer some concept of the file's contents relative to other files. The file name should be less than or equal to 64 characters including the appropriate file extension. You should use only letters (lowercase), numbers, or hyphens in the name. You should not use blank spaces. When naming files, it is important to remember that—to avoid truncation—the length of the entire path of the file should not exceed 230 characters.

O. Naming Folders

The terms *folder* and *subfolder* are used in this guidance and are intended to be synonymous with *directory* and *subdirectory*. The main submission, regional administrative folders, and certain subfolders should have specific names for proper and efficient processing of the submission. Recommendations regarding naming the main submission folders and regional administrative folders can be found in Section III, below. Other specific folder names can be found in the specifications associated with this guidance. You can use only letters (lower case), numbers, or hyphens in the name. You should not use blank spaces. The length of the folder name should not exceed 64 characters. When naming folders, it is important to remember that the length of the entire path should not exceed 230 characters. You should not include empty folders in the submission.

P. File Formats

We recommend that you send electronic documents in the file formats specified in this guidance. We will not be able to manage, process, archive, or review documents provided in other file formats.

The following file formats should be used:

- PDF for reports and forms
- SAS XPORT (version 5) transport files (XPT) for datasets
- ASCII text files (e.g., SAS program files, NONMEM control files) using *txt* for the file extension
- XML for documents, data, and document information files
- Stylesheets (XSL) and document type definition (DTD) for the XML document information files
- Microsoft Word for draft labeling (because Microsoft Word can change, check our Web site for the current version)

In the future, we may consider other electronic file formats for use with electronic submissions, or we may consider the use of the current formats with other electronic submissions. We intend to publish guidance to advise on the use of file formats for specific types of submissions for use in the future.

Q. PDF Bookmarks and Hypertext Links

For documents with a table of contents, provide bookmarks and hypertext links for each item listed in the table of contents including tables, figures, publications, references, and associated appendices. These bookmarks and hypertext links are essential for efficient navigation through documents. You should make the bookmark hierarchy identical to the table of contents. Navigation efficiency is also improved by providing hypertext links throughout the body of the document to supporting annotations, related sections, references, appendices, tables, or figures that are not located on the same page.

It is possible to link to other documents in a submission using relative paths when creating hypertext linking. Absolute links that reference specific drives and root directories are not functional once the submission is loaded onto the document repository. For example, the link path ../../../123456/0001/.. will work, but the link c:1234560001... will not work. However, you should keep in mind that some documents may be subsequently replaced or appended, possibly rendering the link obsolete, so linking should be used cautiously.

When creating bookmarks and hypertext links, choose the magnification setting *Inherit Zoom* so that the destination page displays at the same magnification level that the reviewer is using for the rest of the document.

R. Sending Electronic Submissions

All submissions provided in electronic format must be sent to the appropriate central document room facility for processing to maintain the integrity of the submission as required under 21 CFR part 11. Electronic documents sent directly to division document rooms or to reviewers bypass the controls established for the receipt and archiving of documents and are not considered official documents for review. See the associated specifications for more information, including electronic transmission.

S. Technical Problems or Questions

If you have any questions on technical issues related to providing electronic submissions according to the recommendations in this guidance, contact the electronic submission coordinator at esub@cder.fda.gov. Specific technical issues related to submissions to CBER should be sent to esubprep@cber.fda.gov. Specific questions pertaining to content should be directed to the appropriate review division or office.

III. ORGANIZING THE MAIN SUBMISSION FOLDER

All documents in the electronic submission should be placed in a main submission folder using a four-digit sequence number for the application with the original submission for an application designated 0000. You should assign numbers for each submission to the same application with consecutive numbers. For example, the folder for the 3rd submission to an application, whether it is an amendment, supplement, or general correspondence is numbered 0002. The 4th submission is numbered 0003. This also applies to applications where previous submissions were not based on the ICH eCTD specifications. For example, if the submission is the 25th and the previous 24 were in paper, you would number the folder 0024. You should place the eCTD backbone file for modules 2 to 5 for the submission in this folder (*index.xml*). You should place the checksum file (e.g., index-md5.txt) in the same folder. Sequence numbers are used to differentiate between submissions for the same application and do not need to correspond to the order they are received by the Agency.

We recommend that you use subfolders to organize files in a submission, including for each module *m1*, *m2*, *m3*, *m4*, and *m5*, respectively. There is a subfolder *util* to organize eCTD technical files in the submission. Place these subfolders in the sequence number folder (e.g., folder named 0000 for the initial submission to an application). Do not include empty subfolders.

The following sections provide guidance for organizing the folders and files in the *m1*, *m2*, *m3*, *m4*, *m5*, and *util* folders. In addition, you can find instructions on preparing the submission of an electronic application to CBER at http://www.fda.gov/cber/esub/esub.htm.

A. Module 1 Administrative Information and Prescribing Information Folder

Module 1 contains administrative and labeling documents. The organization of the documents in module 1 is the same for all applications and related submissions. The subject matter for each document should be assigned to the lowest level of the hierarchy outlined in the associated document "Comprehensive Table of Contents Headings and Hierarchy." Note that some headings apply only to specific applications or specific submissions. You should create a folder named *us* and place it in the folder named *m1*. The documents for module 1 should be placed in the *us* folder including the *us-regional.xml* file pertaining to the eCTD backbone files for module 1. Below are some additional details on providing specific types of documents.

1. eCTD Backbone Document Information Files. The details on creating this file are in the associated document "eCTD Backbone Files Specification for Module 1."

2. Cover Letter (Optional). If you decide to include a cover letter, we recommend you include the following information:

- Description of the submission including appropriate regulatory information
- Description of the submission including the approximate size of the submission (e.g., 2 gigabytes), the format used for DLT tapes, and the type and number of electronic media used (e.g., three CDROMs), if applicable
- Statement that the submission is virus free with a description of the software (name, version, and company) used to check the files for viruses
- Regulatory and technical point of contact for the submission

3. Labeling. The following section describes how to provide specific labeling documents.

    a. Labeling History. You can provide a history summarizing labeling changes as a single PDF file. The following information will help us confirm changes made to the labeling:

- Complete list of the labeling changes being proposed in the current submission and the explanation for the changes.
- Date of the last approved labeling.
- History of all changes since the last approved labeling. With each change, you should note the submission that originally described the change and the explanation for the change.
- List of supplements pending approval that may affect the review of the labeling in the current submission.

    b. Content of Labeling. See the guidance for industry on *Providing Regulatory Submissions in Electronic Format—Content of Labeling* for details on providing the content of labeling files.

    c. Labeling Samples. Each labeling sample (e.g., carton labels, container labels, package inserts) should be provided as individual PDF files. The samples should (1) include all panels, if applicable; (2) be provided in their actual size; and (3) reflect the actual color proposed for use.

4. Advertisements and Promotional Material. Advertisements and promotional labeling include material submitted under 21 CFR 314.81(b)(3)(i) or 601.12(f)(4) as part of the postmarketing reporting regulations for approved applications, submitted under the requirements of 21 CFR 314.550 and 601.45 (part of the accelerated approval requirements and restricted distribution for drug and biological products), or voluntarily submitted to INDs. You should submit promotional material to the appropriate application. You should not mix submissions of advertisements and promotional labeling with submissions containing other types of information.

    Each promotional piece should be provided as an individual PDF file. In cases when promotional writing or images cover more than one page (e.g., a brochure spread), the reviewer should be able to view the entire layout at one time. For three-dimensional objects, you should provide a digital image of the object in sufficient detail to allow us to review the promotional material. In addition, you should provide information adequate to determine the size of the object (e.g., point size, dimensions). A dimensional piece shown flat, such as a flattened carton, can also be submitted.

If you choose to include cover letters with your submissions of advertising and promotional material, they should be provided as individual PDF files and indicate for the reviewer any additional important information, such as which materials need priority reviews.

If references are provided, each reference should be submitted as an individual PDF file and placed in the appropriate module based on subject matter. If possible, you should highlight the sections of the full reference that you refer to in the promotional materials. When a reference is used to support a claim in proposed promotional materials voluntarily submitted for advisory opinion or Agency comment, you should provide a hypertext link to the page of the reference or labeling that contains the supporting information.

For promotional materials submitted as part of the postmarketing reporting requirements, you may choose to provide hypertext links to references or labeling. References improve the efficiency of a review.

5.   Marketing Annual Reports.   In the postmarketing study commitments files, you should include a bookmark for each study described.

6.   Information Amendments.   You should include documents that are provided in information amendments in the appropriate module using the appropriate headings to describe the subject matter. In the unusual case when information amendments do not fit appropriately under any heading in the CTD, you should place the documents in module 1 under the heading "Information Amendment: Information Not Covered Under Modules 2 to 5." You should provide a separate PDF file for each subject covered. Documents that apply to more than one module should be placed under the heading "Multiple Module Information Amendments."

B.   Module 2 Summary Folder

You should place the documents for module 2 in the *m2* folder. The subject matter for each document should be specific for the lowest level of the hierarchy outlined in the associated document "Comprehensive Table of Contents Headings and Hierarchy." Each document should be provided as an individual PDF file. The subfolders described in the *M2 eCTD: Electronic Common Technical Document Specification* are not necessary for the review of the submission. If you choose to use the additional subfolder, we will maintain the subfolder structure so links will function properly.

C.   Module 3 Quality Folder

The organization of the module 3 folder is the same for all applications and related submissions. You should place the documents for module 3 in the *m3* folder. The subject matter for each document should be specific for the lowest level of the hierarchy outlined in the associated document "Comprehensive Table of Contents Headings and Hierarchy." Each document should be provided as an individual PDF file. The subfolders described in the *M2 eCTD: Electronic Common Technical Document Specification* are not necessary for the review of the submission. If you choose to use the additional subfolder, we will maintain the subfolder structure used so links will function properly.

You should provide the files pertaining to Key Literature References (CTD Section 3.3) as individual PDF files. The filenames should be short and meaningful.

D. Module 4 Safety Folder

The organization of the module 4 folder is the same for all applications and related submissions. You should place the documents for module 4 in the *m4* folder. The subject matter for each document should be specific for the lowest level of the hierarchy outlined in the associated document "Comprehensive Table of Contents Headings and Hierarchy." The headings for study reports should also be specific for the lowest level of the hierarchy. Each document should be provided as an individual PDF file. The subfolders described in the *M2 eCTD: Electronic Common Technical Document Specification* are not necessary for the review of the submission. If you choose to use the additional subfolder, we will maintain the subfolder structure so links will function properly.

1. Study Reports.   Typically, a single document should be provided for each study report included in this module. However, if you provide the study reports as multiple documents, you should confine the subject matter of each document to a single item in the following list.

- Synopsis
- Study report body
- Protocol and amendments
- Signatures of principal or coordinating investigator(s)
- Audit certificates and reports
- Documentation of statistical methods and interim analysis plans
- Documentation of interlaboratory standardization methods of quality assurance procedures if used
- Publications based on the study
- Important publications referenced in the report
- Compliance and/or drug concentration data
- Individual subject data listings
  - —Data tabulations
    - —Data tabulations datasets
    - —Data definitions
  - —Data listing
    - —Data listing datasets
    - —Data definitions
  - —Analysis datasets
    - —Analysis datasets
    - —Analysis programs
    - —Data definitions
  - —IND safety reports

In the following examples, you should provide the study reports as separate documents:

- Documents previously submitted. If you have provided a document in a previous submission (e.g., protocol), you should provide a reference to the protocol, not resubmit the protocol.

- Additional information added. If you think you will want to add information to the study report over time (e.g., audit information, publication based on the study), you should provide the study reports as separate documents and then the new information can be provided as a separate file, rather than replacing the entire study report.

- Different file formats. If you submit the individual animal data listings as datasets (e.g., SAS transport files), you should provide these as separate files from the study reports (e.g., submitted as PDF files).

When providing a study report, you should include the study tagging file (STF) described in the associated document "The eCTD Backbone File Specifcation for Study Tagging Files."

2. Literature References. You should provide each literature reference as an individual PDF file. The filenames should be short and meaningful.

3. Datasets. See the associated document "Study Data Specifications" for details on providing datasets and related files (e.g., data definition file, program files).

E. Module 5 Clinical Study Reports Folder

The organization of the module 5 folder is the same for all applications and related submissions. You should place the documents for module 5 in the *m5* folder. The subject matter for each document should be specific for the lowest level of the hierarchy outlined in the associated document "Comprehensive Table of Contents Headings and Hierarchy." One exception is that legacy study reports can be provided as a single document. Each document should be provided as an individual PDF file. The subfolders described in the guidance *M2 eCTD: Electronic Common Technical Document Specification* are not necessary for the review of the submission. If you choose to use the additional subfolder, we will maintain the subfolder structure so links will function properly.

1. Tabular Listing of All Clinical Studies. You should provide the tabular listing of all clinical studies as a single PDF file.

2. Study Reports. Typically, clinical study reports are provided as more than one document based on the ICH E3 guidance document when providing a study.[9] In addition, if you have provided a document in a previous submission (e.g., protocol), you should provide a reference to the protocol rather than resubmitting the protocol. In cases when a legacy report has already been prepared as a single electronic document, you can provide

---

[9] When providing a study report, you should include the study tagging file (STF) described in the associated document "The eCTD Backbone File Specification for Study Tagging Files."

the entire study report, other than the case report forms (CRFs) and individual data listings, as a single document. The individual documents that should be included in a study report are listed below:

- Synopsis[10] (E3 2)
- Study report (E3 1, 3 to 15)
- Protocol and amendments (E3 16.1.1)
- Sample case report forms (E3 16.1.2)
- List of IECs or IRBs (E3 16.1.3) and consent forms
- List and description of investigators (E3 16.1.4) and sites
- Signatures of principal or coordinating investigator(s) or sponsor's responsible medical officer (E3 16.1.5)
- Listing of patients receiving test drug(s) from specified batch (E3 16.1.6)
- Randomizations scheme (E3 16.1.7)
- Audit certificates (E3 16.1.8) and reports
- Documentation of statistical methods (E3 16.1.9) and interim analysis plans
- Documentation of interlaboratory standardization methods of quality assurance procedures if used (E3 16.1.10)
- Publications based on the study (E3 16.1.11)
- Important publications referenced in the report (E3 16.1.12)
- Discontinued patients (E3 16.2.1)
- Protocol deviations (E3 16.2.2)
- Patients excluded from the efficacy studies (E3 16.2.3)
- Demographic data (E3 16.2.4)
- Compliance and/or drug concentration data (E3 16.2.5)
- Individual efficacy response data (E3 16.2.6)
- Adverse event listings (E3 16.2.7)
- Listing of individual laboratory measurements by patient (E3 16.2.8)
- Case report forms (E3 16.3)
- Individual patient data listings (CRTs) (E3 16.4)
  - —Data tabulations
    - —Data tabulations datasets
    - —Data definitions
    - —Annotated case report form
  - —Data listing
    - —Data listing datasets
    - —Data definitions
    - —Annotated case report form

---

[10] The synopsis should be provided as a document separate from the study report.

—Analysis datasets
    —Analysis datasets
    —Analysis programs
    —Data definitions
    —Annotated case report form
—Subject profiles
—IND safety reports

3. Case Report Forms. You should provide an individual subject's complete CRF as a single PDF file. If a paper CRF was used in the clinical trial, the electronic CRF should be a scanned image of the paper CRF including all original entries with all modifications, addenda, corrections, comments, annotations, and any extemporaneous additions. If electronic data capture was used in the clinical trial, you should submit a PDF-generated form or other PDF representation of the information (e.g., subject profile).

You should use the subject's unique identifier as the title of the document and the file name. These names are used to assist reviewers in finding the CRF for an individual subject. Each CRF must have bookmarks as part of the comprehensive table of contents required under 21 CFR 314.50(b). We recommend bookmarks for each CRF domain and study visit to help the reviewer navigate the CRFs. For addenda and corrections, making a hypertext link from the amended item to the corrected page or addendum is a useful way to avoid confusion. Bookmarks for these items should be displayed at the bottom of the hierarchy.

4. Datasets. See the associated document "Study Data Specifications" for details on providing datasets and related files (e.g., data definition files, program files). For subject profiles, you should use the subject's unique identifier in the title of the document and the file name.

5. Periodic Safety Update Reports. To facilitate electronic submissions, we have divided the postmarketing periodic adverse drug experience report into three parts: (1) individual case safety reports (ICSRs), (2) ICSR attachments, if applicable, and (3) descriptive information. The descriptive information includes the narrative summary and analysis of the information in the report (i.e., periodic ICSRs and ICSR attachments), an analysis of the 15-day alert reports submitted during the reporting interval (i.e., expedited ICSRs and ICSR attachments), and the history of actions taken since the last report because of adverse drug experiences (e.g., labeling changes, studies initiated) as described in 21 CFR 314.80(c)(2)(ii)(a) and (c) and 600.80(c)(2)(ii)(A) and (C)). You should supply the descriptive information as an individual PDF file. You should provide bookmarks for each of the sections and subsections of this report. ICSR and ICSR attachments should be provided as described in the guidance for industry *Providing Regulatory Submissions in Electronic Format—Postmarketing Periodic Adverse Drug Experience Reports.*

6. Literature References. You should provide each literature reference as an individual PDF file. The filenames should be short and meaningful.

IV. UTILITY FOLDER

You should create two folders, *dtd* and *style*, and place them in the *util* folder.

A. Document-Type Definition Folder

You should place the document-type definition (DTD) that you used to create the eCTD backbone file (regional.xml), the DTD you used to create the FDA Regional eCTD backbone file (us-index.xml), and the DTD used for the STF in the folder named *dtd*. You should use the most recent DTD.[11]

B. Style Folder

You should use the most recent stylesheet. See the guidance for industry *M2 eCTD: Electronic Common Technical Document Specification.*

---

[11] See the FDA Web site at http://www.fda.gov/cder/regulatory/ersr/.

CHAPTER 7

EMEA/FDA COORDINATION

7.1 INTRODUCTION

Reconciling the requirements of the FDA and the EMEA can be a headache for large, well-established medical device, pharmaceutical, food, and biotech organizations and can be a matter of survival for early-stage companies on a short financial leash. It's a delicate balance: Companies neither want to maintain expensive and burdensome dual systems for meeting the requirements of both agencies, nor do they want to underinvest to the point that their investigational new drugs are rejected by either.

Fundamental philosophical and stylistic differences between the US Food and Drug Administration (FDA) and the European Union European Medicines Agency (EMEA) cause many companies to adopt a regulatory strategy for treating submissions and compliance issues of these two agencies in unnecessarily expensive (or market limiting) ways. Some companies set up parallel entities in the United States and Europe to work independently, coping with their respective agencies in isolation. Other entities select one of the two agencies for primacy and deal with the second sequentially, losing revenue opportunity and valuable time. Still other organizations focus exclusively on either the EU or US market, in effect surrendering the nonselected market. None of these self-limiting strategies is necessary: It is possible to cost effectively bridge the gap between FDA and EMEA policies, and cope with both simultaneously by taking advantage of the significant overlap in their regulations and approaches.

The FDA's July 2008 release of "Guidance for Industry: cGMP for Phase 1 Investigational New Drugs" (cGMP1), whose EMEA counterpart is "Good Automated Manufacturing Practices, Version 5 (GAMP5)," points up the dilemma anew. In the absence of an explicit harmonization document, the best approach to the problem is to (1) understand the philosophical differences between the two agencies, (2) examine the differences in the documents in light of those philosophical differences, and (3) consider the most promising avenue for reconciling them: Quality by Design (QbD).

Cost-Contained Regulatory Compliance: For the Pharmaceutical, Biologics, and Medical Device Industries, First Edition. Sandy Weinberg.
© 2011 John Wiley & Sons, Inc. Published 2011 by John Wiley & Sons, Inc.

7.2   PHILOSOPHY: SAFETY VERSUS ACCESS

To some extent, all regulatory agencies are involved in a dynamic tension between competing and often incompatible goals. The EMEA and the FDA are charged by their respective governments to both assure public access to drugs and assure the safety of those drug products. If the agency focuses on maximizing the public's access to potentially beneficial drugs, it adheres to a policy of promotion, helping to ease the approval and testing process. If, on the other hand, safety is the agency's primary focus, it tends to restrict access by maximizing pre-release analysis and testing.

For historical, legal, and political reasons, the FDA has traditionally emphasized safety (resulting in a relatively small, but presumably safe, pharmacopeia), while the EMEA has tended to maximize access, allowing patients and their physicians greater flexibility in making their own determinations of safety. As a result, the EMEA is generally seen by the industry as cooperative, helping to get drugs to market, while the FDA is often viewed as obstructionist, reducing access in the name of safety.

Not surprisingly then, the EMEA focuses on the final drug product as tested in Phase 1 (and other phases), while the FDA spends considerable energy and regulatory capital examining the API and raw materials that precede the final product. In effect, the EMEA tests for purity, while the FDA audits and back-traces for the same assurances. In other words, the EMEA emphasizes the end product, and the FDA emphasizes the process.

7.3   CRITICAL DIFFERENCES

This fundamental philosophic difference between the two agencies—a focus on access and end product at the EMEA versus safety and process at FDA—helps account for some important differences between GAMP5 and cGMP1 in three critical areas: requirements for validation, QA/QC policy, and process monitoring.

The GAMP5 guidelines have "automated" built into the name and the philosophy—they envision process and system (computer) validation as integrated entities. An automated process is tested with an Installation Qualification, Operational Qualification, and Performance Qualification to be certain that the automated procedure has been properly installed, tested, and employed.

By contrast, the FDA's cGMP1 document assumes a manual process with only tangential reference to the reality of automated process systems (covered by the FDA in a separate document, 21 CFR Part 11, which defines system validation and provides guidelines for it). In keeping with the agencies' philosophical differences, the EMEA stresses the "bottom line" performance, while the FDA stresses the process itself (procedurally and with automation). Under GAMP5, a Phase 1 investigator would validate the results of an automated analysis system as a functioning analytical unit. Under cGMP1, an investigator would validate the analytical process and, perhaps, depending on risk, separately validate the analytical system that conducts the procedure.

Similarly, the EMEA focuses on Quality Assurance—the general overview questions—regarding a study: Does it produce a reliable result with appropriate quality oversight? While still emphasizing QA, the FDA approach puts equal weight on the Quality Control process, including all aspects of production and operation as well as the final QA overview. The EMEA would potentially rely more heavily on a final quarantine and testing for the release procedure, while the FDA would augment it with step-by-step reviews of the manufacturing and clinical testing plan.

As for process monitoring, the EMEA GAMP5 deemphasizing of process differs significantly from the FDA's Process Analytical Technology (PAT) initiative. Potentially, PAT provides near-continuous and self-correcting cybernetic monitoring of a procedure, method, practice, or course of action. The result again is greater reliance at the FDA on analysis at all phases, with a contrary reliance at EMEA on the final result rather than the interim steps that lead to that result—in short, process understanding versus process outcome.

7.4   THE PATH TO HARMONIZATION: QBD

The FDA's PAT initiative is just the first of three components of Quality by Design, a rigorously science-based approach to drug safety. QbD integrates an understanding of design space, a risk-based approach to compliance, and PAT monitoring. Together, those three elements can help satisfy both the results-focused outlook of the EMEA and the process-focused outlook of the FDA:

- "Design space" is defined in ICH Q8 as "the multi-dimensional combination and interaction of input variables (e.g., material attributes) and process parameters that have been demonstrated to provide assurance of quality."[1] Successfully defining the design space means achieving a full understanding of the various permutations of input variables and process parameters that assure an in-specification product. Design-space analysis establishes flexible operating parameters within which fluctuations are permitted, thus satisfying the FDA's emphasis on Quality Control.

- A full understanding of the multiple, complex interactions among variables makes it possible to predict the outcome from particular permutations. It is then possible to assure an acceptably low risk of failing to achieve the desired clinical attributes, thus opening the way for a risk-based approach to compliance.

- PAT's continuous and cybernetic monitoring of process parameters automates process control, satisfying EMEA's emphasis on testing and Quality Assurance.

Thus QbD promises to effectively harmonize the safety goals of the FDA with the access goals of the EMEA, without compromising either.

Even more promisingly, QbD can ultimately satisfy the QA bent of the EMEA and the QC emphasis of the FDA in a way that improves both. The ability to design-in product and performance characteristics from the first rather than deriving them through testing after the fact more efficiently meets EMEA's results and testing-focused requirements. Meanwhile, the analysis of design space satisfies the FDA's

[1] ICH Harmonized Tripartite Guideline: Pharmaceutical Development Q8, Current *Step 4* version, November 10, 2005, p. 11.

thirst for process understanding, while avoiding cumbersome refilings every time a process parameter is changed. Biotechs that adopt QbD will not only be able to meet the differing EMEA and FDA requirements, but do so in a way that could significantly lighten their regulatory burden.

7.5 STRATEGY FOR SUBMISSIONS

If the goal is to minimize duplicated effort and to streamline the processes of making regulatory submissions (IND, NDA, etc.) to both FDA and EMEA, strategic decisions are complicated by tactical requirements for formatting and style. But while these logistical requirements vary significantly between the agencies, the actual content requirements of the submissions are remarkably similar. By treating the two submissions with overlapping variations on the same project, it is possible to significantly reduce the combined cost of preparation. Unfortunately, many companies either prepare their US and European submissions separately using parallel teams or using a sequential submissions strategy.

To minimize the costs associated with a simultaneous submission to both the FDA and EMEA, begin by developing modules describing, including, and interpreting the evidence in support of the key issues related to the regulatory questions. For example, develop a module demonstrating the integrity (or control of) the blood–brain barrier; a module demonstrating the efficacy of the drug, device, or biologic in excess of placebo effects; the purity of the food, pharmaceutical, or biological product; and so forth.

While the specific nature and number of regulatory questions will vary with the type of submission and the categorization of the product, they can generally be delineated in pre-submissions conferences or gleaned from regulatory guidance documents.[2] Once listed, a module should be prepared for each individual question.

Preparing a submission for EMEA and for FDA is then a matter of carefully following the formatting requirements of each agency; selecting the appropriate modules for the regulatory questions relevant to the specific agency; and plugging those modules into the appropriate location in the submissions format. Most modules will be included in both applications, generally in different orders and occasionally with differing introductions, but the costs associated with preparing both submissions simultaneously should be a fraction of separate or sequential preparations.

7.6 STRATEGY FOR COMPLIANCE

The FDA conducts facility inspections both within the United States and in the European Union (and other regions); the EMEA conducts inspection visits in EU countries, and reviews the results of FDA inspections. Both agencies are seeking confirmation of compliance with self-regulation, focusing largely on internal quality assurance and control.

---

[2] See Weinberg, S. *Guidebook to Drug Regulatory Submissions*, John Wiley & Sons, Hoboken, NJ, 2009.

There are four basic steps in maximizing simultaneous (and hence cost-effective) compliance in anticipation of FDA and EMEA visits: training, outside audits, translation services, and indexed SOPs.

First, provide extensive training for all relevant personnel in the methods of coping with a regulatory inquiry and investigation. These strategies include:

- Seeking clarification in advance of answering, particularly when dealing with linguistic complexities. At a recent audit in Puerto Rico, an FDA investigator was prepared to cite a company for a major infraction when the plant manager replied to a routine inquiry that no SOPs were in use. The problem was averted when, in response to a clarifying question, the manager explained that they relied on the use of "POS" guidelines: the Spanish translation of Standard Operating Procedures!

- Answering exactly what is asked. Too many times an inspection is sent off track when a response ranges wide of the actual question. "Where do you archive data?" does not need to focus on the methods of storage, the recovery times, or the results of the last restoration drill.

- Finding the right respondee. A response of "let me find the proper person to provide that answer" is perfectly acceptable. Well-written Standard Operating Procedures will quickly identify the appropriate person to respond to specific questions.

Second, consider using a credible, independent auditor to preempt the regulatory visit. In many cases a thorough report written by a credentialed auditor and tied to specific (FDA and EMEA) regulations will satisfy an investigator. The investigator will review the report, examine the credentials of the auditor, and generally move to other issues or facilities. Chapter 2 provided some guidance about the kinds of credentials required and the regulatory standards to be followed.

Third, consider formal adoption of a standard language for the entire company (generally English is selected) and have all documents translated into that language. If multiple languages are to be used (often to assure understanding of SOPs by local personnel) or if the language selected in not English, have translations available for FDA investigators. While translated documents are not legally required, they will ease the process with unilingual FDA people. Some EMEA documents[3] require multilingual applications, but English is prominently included in the list (along with French, German, Italian, Icelandic, Finnish, and others). Having English language documents available, either as primary documents or translations, will generally satisfy both FDA and EMEA visitors.

Finally, cross index all SOPs (and related documents) to appropriate sections of both the FDA's cGMPs and the EMEA's GAMP4/5 regulations. An SOP for periodic review of automated audit trails in software systems can be tied to the specific sections of 21 CFR Part 11 (FDA) and to the GAMP4 Requirements (EMEA).[4] This cross indexing—generally a record adjacent to the versioning notation on each

---

[3] Orphan Drug Applications, for example.
[4] See Chapter 12.

SOP—provides the ability to demonstrate compliance with both agency's guidelines and also acts as a control to make certain that all required regulatory documents are referenced in appropriate SOP.

These four strategies can provide a strong frame for both FDA and EMEA compliance and can cost-effectively permit a company to approach compliance issues in tandem rather than sequentially.

Incidentally, some international companies have successfully extended these concepts to regulations in Australia, Switzerland, Brazil, and (with some difficulty) Japan.

7.7 CLINICAL RESEARCH

An additional cost-containment strategy can help control expenses if opting from joint FDA and EMEA simultaneous jurisdiction: the design and use of common clinical research studies in support of an ANDA, NDA, BLA, or Medical Device PMA.

Carefully designed clinical research conducted in the United States or in EU Europe (or, for that matter, anywhere else) can be submitted as effective supporting evidence to both the FDA and the EMEA. While the regulations of the two agencies differ in philosophy and format, their content is effectively, if unofficially, harmonized.

To minimize costs and maximize joint applicability, the FDA's Critical Path guidelines will serve effectively.[5] The guidelines provide generalized models for conducting clinical research, closely (if accidentally) harmonized between FDA and EMEA approaches. Following these plans, along with the professional standards of effective double-blinded clinical studies, should produce data acceptable to both agencies.

To assure this acceptability, clinical sites and data collection/analysis procedures should be visited by either representatives of FDA and EMEA, or by a qualified independent auditor. Approval criteria will include quality assurance oversight of the clinical testing process, and confirmation of conformity to the Investigator's Brochure and study design.

At least in theory, the same kind of quality assurance oversight is provided by the peer review process of major journals. The FDA therefore has established a mechanism for cited published studies conducted by outside researchers as support for a new drug application. This provision is the 505(b)2 process, a controversial procedure to permit submissions of NDAs partially or entirely supported by independent, published studies. While the EMEA has not established a separate and defined process, it too accepts published studies as support for a clinical research submission.

The FDA's 505(b)2 process and its parallel EMEA acceptance of published studies in support of applications provides an opportunity to use a third-party inde-

---

[5] See von Eshenbach, Andrew C., MD. Statement to the Senate Agriculture, Rural Development, Food and Drug Administration, and Related Agencies Appropriations Sub-Committee, July 2007.

pendent entity—referrer and prestigious international journals—as a common source of supporting documentation. Studies conducted by the applying company, by outside academic teams, or by outside researchers with financial or technical support from the applying company can provide published evidence credible to both the FDA and EMEA, thereby allowing simultaneous and cost-contained dual applications.

7.8 SUMMARY

While the FDA and EMEA have significantly differing regulatory philosophies and rely on related but separate core guidance documents, it is possible to replace strategies of sequential, parallel, or single target submissions with a much more cost-effective simultaneous dual application. In similar fashion, common strategies for compliance and for clinical research can lead to efficient and effective joint dealings with the difference agencies.

Three specific approaches are suggested. For submissions, organize data into modules defined by research-related regulatory questions. When using the format and stylistic requirements of each agency, plug in the appropriate module in the application section as required. The differences between FDA and EMEA requirements are largely cosmetic: In almost all cases the same modules will effectively meet the differing regulatory submission requirements.

For compliance, rely heavily on in-house or credible outside auditors to preempt regulatory visits. Use the FDA's Systems Inspection approach, and provide clear audit reports against established standards, with credible compliance documentation. Both agencies will respect this approach and will focus their visits on testing the veracity of the audit reports.

For clinical research, use the FDA's 505(b)2 strategy to maximize the use of outside published research studies in support of applications. In addition, use outside auditors or invited FDA/EMEA visitors to boost the credibility of studies intended for joint FDA and EMEA review.

With these three families of strategies in place, it should be possible to effectively manage simultaneous and significantly overlapping FDA and EMEA regulatory affairs without the need for parallel organizations or delays in the development of supporting documentation.

APPENDIX TO CHAPTER 7

Continuing through painfully slow FDA–EMEA negotiations are likely to cause some revision in standards over time. The following document, supplemented by the US GMP auditing checklist, should provide the necessary detailed guidance to permit implementation of this cost-containment strategy.

US GMP AUDIT CHECKLIST

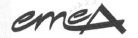

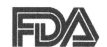

European Agency for the Evaluation of Medicinal Products	European Commission	US Food and Drug Administration

MEDICINES REGULATION: TRANSATLANTIC ADMINISTRATIVE SIMPLIFICATION ACTION PLAN

Introduction

Under the auspices of the Transatlantic Economic Council, on 28 November 2007 the European Commission hosted the Transatlantic Administrative Simplification Workshop which was co-chaired by the European Commission and the United States (US) Food and Drug Administration (FDA) and organised in collaboration with the European Medicines Agency (EMEA) and the Heads of the EU National Medicines Agencies (HMA). The key objective was to identify opportunities for administrative simplification through transatlantic cooperation at the level of administrative practices and guidelines. The key guiding principles for the proposals were as follows:

- No change to legislation should be required.
- The simplifications should maintain or increase current levels of public health protection.

During the workshop, industry presented a diverse range of proposals for administrative simplification through transatlantic and international collaboration and harmonization. The

Cost-Contained Regulatory Compliance: For the Pharmaceutical, Biologics, and Medical Device Industries, First Edition. Sandy Weinberg.
© 2011 John Wiley & Sons, Inc. Published 2011 by John Wiley & Sons, Inc.

proposals were presented in four thematic panels [on (1) quality and inspections, (2) pharmacovigilance, (3) scientific collaboration, (4) guidelines, format harmonization and electronic submission].

Deliverables

Relieving unnecessary burdens of administrative practices through a careful selection of simplification projects proposed at the workshop could allow more human and fiscal resources to be focused by the industry on greater innovation and efficiency in development of quality products and thereby to greater access to these products by patient populations on both sides of the Atlantic.

FDA contact:
Michelle Limoli
Office of International Programs
  US Food and Drug
  Administration

EC contact:
Matus Ferech
Pharmaceuticals Unit F2, DG
  Enterprise and Industry, European
  Commission

Within the framework of the Workshop, it was agreed that the next steps in the transatlantic administrative simplification process would be careful public health, legal, and practical consideration of the proposals by the EU and US regulators with a view to making public a joint action plan for administrative simplification. Actions should be carried out, either:

- through bilateral work (e.g., under the existing EU–US confidentiality arrangements for medicinal products), or
- through multilateral work (e.g., through the International Conference on Harmonization—ICH)

The Medicines Regulation Transatlantic Administrative Simplification Action Plan is an agreed action plan between the European Commission DG Enterprise and Industry and the United States Food and Drug Administration. On the EU side the Action Plan involves collaboration with the European Medicines Agency and the national medicines agencies of the EEA Member States.

The parties have agreed the following administrative simplification projects:

Project Title	Note
Collaboration on inspections	The Commission/EMEA and the FDA will pilot joint inspections of companies manufacturing pharmaceuticals in the United States and in the EU and of companies manufacturing active pharmaceutical ingredients in third countries.
Collaboration on 3rd country inspection	The Commission/EMEA and the FDA will pilot the exchange of inspection schedules, results, and information on inspected manufacturing sites in order to attain more GMP inspection coverage collectively and to better identify manufacturing sites producing active pharmaceutical ingredients in third countries.

Project Title	Note
Dedicated facilities for high-risk products	The Commission/EMEA and the FDA will step up collaboration to determine to what extent dedicated production facilities are necessary for certain pharmaceuticals taking into account a risk based approach. Subsequently, it is expected that a revised EU guideline will be published for public consultation in the first quarter of 2009. FDA is also in the process of clarifying this issue through proposing amendments to existing regulations and draft guidances that are in the process for issuance.
Biomarkers	The EMEA and the FDA have recently announced successes in their transatlantic work on biomarker development and joint validation for various product development purposes. Both parties will continue to work on this initiative with a view to further biomarker development and joint validation.
Regulatory collaboration on the outputs of the Critical Path and Innovative Medicines Initiatives	EMEA and FDA will exchange assessments of the outputs of the Critical Path and Innovative Medicines Initiatives relevant to medicines regulation and will report findings to the 2009 EC/EMEA/FDA Bilateral meeting.
Combating counterfeit medicines	In addition to the collaborative work with the WHO IMPACT initiative, the Commission and FDA will exchange information on future requirements for track and trace and authentication systems. Commission/EMEA and FDA will exchange information on specific cases of counterfeits.
Collaboration on product-specific Risk Management	Under the EC/EMEA/FDA confidentiality arrangements, the EMEA and FDA will intensify bilateral discussion on proposed specific risk management initiatives for specific new medicinal products and report to the 2009 EC/EMEA/FDA Bilateral meeting.
Convergence of Risk Management formats	The EU and US pharmaceutical industry are invited to conduct a study to compare the EU and US approaches to risk management formats (e.g., E2E, Volume 9a RMP Guidance, REMS, etc.) and to identify opportunities for convergence.
Increasing the uptake of parallel transatlantic scientific advice	Voluntary industry Parallel Scientific Advice for human medicines to be opened to all medicinal products covered by clusters (e.g., pediatrics, oncology, vaccines, pharmacogenomics, orphans). Review of industry uptake and recommendations on procedures by end 2009.
Exchange on Information on herbal medicines	EMEA Committee on Herbal Medicinal Products to provide draft and final monographs to FDA.

Project Title	Note
Collaboration on biosimilar medicinal products/follow on biologicals	EMEA and FDA will compare their experience of biosimilar medicinal products/follow on biologicals and will report to the EC/EMEA/FDA Bilateral meeting by end 2009.
Collaboration on development of medicinal products for children	Under the EC/EMEA/FDA confidentiality arrangements, the EMEA and FDA will intensify bilateral discussion on the development of specific medicinal products for children and will report to the 2009 EC/EMEA/FDA Bilateral meeting.
Convergence in pediatric submissions	In 2009 EC/EMEA will conduct a review of the Commission Pediatric Investigation Plan Guideline, based on experiences to date, with a view to identifying opportunities for transatlantic convergence of submission formats.
Advanced Therapy Medicinal Products	Under the EC/EMEA/FDA confidentiality arrangements, by end 2008, establish a "cluster" on Advanced Therapy Medicinal Products. The cluster to strive for scientific excellence, harmonization of terminology for new technologies and to make recommendations for transatlantic convergence in the administration of regulations for these medicinal products.
Safety reporting from clinical trials	EU/FDA reconfirm their commitment to pursue these topics through ICH.
Harmonization of business rules for single case reports	
Maintenance and updating of the ICH Common Technical Document (CTD)	
Electronic-CTD	

GMP FACILITIES AUDIT CHECKLIST[6]
AUDITING HISTORY COVER SHEET

Facility:

Date(s) of Audit:
Date of Last Audit:
Audit Results Reviewed with/Reported to:
Date:
Follow-Up/Action:
Comments:
Auditor and Date Prepared:

Name:_____
Address _____
Phone:
_____
_____
_____
_____
_____
_____
_____
_____
_____
_____

[6] Formatted with assistance from Ms. Lisa Gonzales, GE Healthcare.

SECTION I: RECEIVING CONTROL

	Response			Reference
	Yes	No	N/A	(21 CFR)
1. Does receiving inspection check incoming shipments to requirements of the purchase order, specifications and applicable drawings?				211.84
2. Do receiving inspection records indicate acceptance or rejection of incoming material?				211.84, 211.184
3. Are material weight checks made upon receipt?				211.84, 211.184 211.101
4. Do receiving inspection records reflect the reasons for rejection?				211.84
5. Are records of receiving materials properly stored?				211.184
6. Are inspected items properly segregated from the material awaiting inspection?				211.42
7. Is inspected material adequately identified as to acceptance or rejection?				211.80
8. Is rejected material adequately controlled?				211.89
9. Are the sampling plans employed by Quality Control sufficient?				211.84

SECTION II: MATERIALS STORAGE AND HANDLING

	Response			Reference
	Yes	No	N/A	(21 CFR)
1. Is access to storerooms and materials storage areas restricted to authorized personnel?				None
2. Are materials handled, identified and stored in a manner that will prevent damage, contamination, mix-up, and/ or loss?				211.80 211.42
3. Are accountability records kept to permit forward and backward traceability?				211.188 211.184
4. Are stocks reinspected and tested at intervals?				211.87
5. Are stocks rotated?				211.86, 211.150
6. Are raw materials and preweighed materials stored off the floor on pallets/shelving to permit cleaning and inspection?				211.80c
7. Is there a sufficient accountability system for labels?				211.125c
8. Are preweighed and original containers of raw materials properly identified; such as in-house code number batch/lot number, product disposition/status and other information required by procedure?				211.80d 211.101b
9. Are raw materials properly identified as to status; approved, rejected, quarantined?				211.80d
10. Are all raw materials approved (released by Quality department) before issued to a batch for use?				211.84e 211.101c
11. Are reject materials identified and segregated from approved materials?				211.42, 211.80 211.89
12. Are raw materials stored under quarantine until examined for released or rejection:				211.82, 211.84 211.89
13. Do raw material records list the identity and quantity of each shipment of each lot, the name of the supplier the receiving in-house lot number, and the date of receipt?				211.84 211.184

SECTION IIIA: PRODUCTION/IN-PROCESS CONTROL, GENERAL

	Response			Reference
	Yes	No	N/A	(21 CFR)
1. Are all employees wearing appropriate clothing including proper head, face and hand coverings?				211.28a
2. Are employees performing their assigned function in an orderly manner, according to instructions and procedures?				211.25a
3. Are there written procedures for production and process control?				211.100a
4. Are procedures being followed?				211.100b
5. Are training records current?				211.25a
6. Does the production equipment appear to be appropriately designed, constructed and maintained?				211.63 211.65 211.67a
7. Are equipment cleaning use logs being maintained?				211.67c 211.82
8. Are procedures for the cleaning, sanitizing, and maintenance of equipment and utensils being followed?				211.67b
9. Are the departmental instructions for general cleaning being followed?				211.56b
10. Are the proper cleaning materials and solutions being prepared and used according to departmental instructions?				211.56b 211.67
11. Are utensils cleaned to prevent contamination between different product usages?				211.67
12. Where appropriate, are containers and utensils that require cleaning, and that are clean, properly identified segregated and stored in appropriate areas?				211.67b 211.105a

SECTION IIIB: PRODUCTION/IN-PROCESS CONTROL, GENERAL

	Response			Reference
	Yes	No	N/A	(21 CFR)
1. Are master and batch production records properly assembled and sufficient in the following content:				211.186 211.188
A. Is each prepared, dated and signed in full signature by one person and independently checked, dated and signed by a second?				211.186 211.188a
B. Are batch records kept at the work stations during operation?				211.100b
C. Have batch records been, or are being completed properly?				211.186a 211.188b
D. Is a complete list of components provided?				211.186(b)(3)
E. Are the weights and measures of each raw material recorded when measured?				211.188(b)(4)
F. Are information and signatures recorded on records immediately after performing an operation?				211.100(b)
G. Are there inventory records for the use of each raw material?				211.184(c)
H. Can a raw material be traced to its use in a particular lot of product?				211.184(c) 211.188(b)(4)
I. Are there records fully documenting any planned or unplanned variances from procedures or operations				211.100(b) 211.192
J. Are raw materials reconciled against each in-house lot number?				211.184(c)
K. Are reconciliation records within established limits?				211.184(c)
L. Have any discrepancies in reconciliation records been investigated and documented?				211.192
M. Are calibrated stickers/tags present and dated on scales and balances?				211.68(a) 211.160(b) 211.194(d)
N. Are scales zeroed before weighing operations?				211.160(b)(4) 211.194(d)
O. Are scales that are not in proper working order identified to prevent use?				211.160(b)(4)

	Response			Reference
	Yes	No	N/A	(21 CFR)
2. Have time limitations on the holding of processing and in-process items been established and are they being adhered to?				211.111
3. Are changes to the issued batch records approved prior to the start of work and documented on the batch records?				211.100
4. Are proper gowning techniques and coverings employed?				211.28
5. Are non-fiber-releasing filters used for liquid filtration in the manufacture of injectable drug products?				211.72
6. Are bagged or boxed components stored off the floor?				211.80
7. Are lubricants and coolants controlled properly such that they cannot come in contact with product containers, closures, in-process materials, or finished products?				211.65(b)
8. Have the sterilization processes been validated?				211.100

SECTION IV: FACILITIES AND METROLOGY

	Response			Reference
	Yes	No	N/A	(21 CFR)
1. Are operations performed in defined areas to prevent contamination and mix-ups?				211.42(b,c)
2. Are production areas sufficient in size, construction, and location?				211.42(a)
3. Does the entire area meet an acceptable level of cleanliness, and are all areas in an orderly condition?				211.42, 211.46 211.56, 211.58 211.67
4. Are appropriate exhaust and vacuum systems employed in operations to minimize air contamination?				211.46
5. Are the air-handling systems operating properly?				211.46(a,b,c)
6. Are all light fixtures operating properly?				211.44
7. Is waste and trash collected and removed when appropriate and are there written SOPs?				211.50 211.56(a,b)
8. Is there no evidence of infestation by rodents, birds, insects, or vermin?				211.56(a)
9. Is there a formal pest control program and are records up to date?				211.56(c)
10. Are maintenance and cleaning logs or records accessible and completed properly?				211.63 211.67(c) 211.182
11. Are there adequate written calibration procedures? Is there a record of the calibrations being performed?				211.68 211.194(d) 211.160(b)(4)
12. Are drains to sewers designed with an air break to prevent back siphonage?				211.48(b)
13. Are the environmental systems adequate to control air pressure, humidity, temperature, microorganisms, and particulate matter?				211.42 211.46
14. Are the adjacent exterior grounds manicured?				211.56

	Response			Reference
	Yes	No	N/A	(21 CFR)
15. Are adequate washing facilities with hot/cold water soap, clean toilets, air driers, or single service towels provided?				211.52
16. Have support systems such as water, vacuum, and compressed air been validated to assure causal variability in the characteristics of in-process material and final product?				211.00
17. Is there a designated area for eating, drinking, and smoking?				211.42
18. Is there an acceptable separate gowning area?				211.42(c)
19. Are the environmental control systems periodically inspected and are such inspections documented?				211.42c(10)IV
20. Are tools, gauges, and test equipment identified to reflect the date calibrated and next calibration date?				211.68
21. Does the calibration data reflect the person responsible for calibration?				211.68
22. Are adequate facilities used for storage of tools gauges and test equipment?				311.68
23. Are the positive atmospheric controls calibrated and monitored?				211.68
24. Are there positive pressure differentials with all doors leading into less clean areas?				211.42c(10)iii
25. Are drawings and blueprints adequately controlled?				211.42

SECTION V: QUALITY CONTROL, FINAL INSPECTION

	Response			Reference
	Yes	No	N/A	(21 CFR)
1. Is there a final inspection performed by Quality Control on a batch by batch basis?				211.22 211.192
2. Does Quality Control have written procedures to assure that production records are reviewed?				211.22(d)
3. Is there a thorough investigation of any discrepancies found during the final review of the production documents?				211.192 211.188(b)(11)
4. Is the product checked for correct expiration dating?				211.137
5. Are records of inspection and test data maintained?				211.160 211.134
6. Are adequate sampling plans used?				211.165
7. Do the sampling procedures specify the manner in which the samples are to be pulled and by whom?				211.160 211.165
8. Is there a classification of defects?				211.16
9. Are reserved samples of finished products maintained?				211.170 211.134
10. Has the accuracy, sensitivity, specificity, and reproducibility of the test methods been demonstrated via validation?				211.165(e)
11. Are the quality control facilities adequate?				211.22
12. Do the facilities have adequate equipment for the performance of Quality Control functions?				211.22 211.42(c)(9)
13. Are all components, manufacturing materials, in-process materials, packaging materials, and labeling tested prior to release to production?				211.184(a)
14. Are test procedures documented?				211.194
15. Are classifications of defects utilized during visual and dimensional inspections?				211.165

	Response			Reference
	Yes	No	N/A	(21 CFR)
16. Are raw material file samples maintained for future reference?				211.84(b)
17. Are laboratory reagents and other chemical supplies identified, tested and expiration dated?				211.194(c)
18. Are laboratory instruments requiring calibration maintained according to the calibration procedures?				211.194(d)
19. Is there a written microbial monitoring program for nonsterile products?				211.113

INTERNAL FACILITY AUDIT CHECKLIST

SECTION VI: QUALITY ASSURANCE

	Response			Reference
	Yes	No	N/A	(21 CFR)
1. Are the responsibilities and procedures applicable to Quality Control documented and approved?				211.22
2. Do written procedures exist governing a document change control system?				211.100
3. Are adequate controls in effect to assure drawings, change notices, and specifications are in use at the time and place of the operation?				211.100
4. Are records maintained which reflect a history of change incorporation?				211.100
5. Are the documents up to date?				211.100
6. Are the documents comprehensive in text?				211.100
7. Are the procedures employed by Quality Assurance documented?				211.22(d)
8. Does Quality assurance have the authority to approve/reject plant equipment, process and procedural changes?				211.22
9. Is an adequate product complaint/product failure handling system in effect and are investigations facilitated properly?				211.198 211.192
10. Is there an adequate stability program?				211.166
11. Is batch record data reviewed on an annual basis to determine continual acceptability of quality standards specifications, manufacturing, and control procedures?				211.180(e)
12. Does Quality Assurance approve/reject product manufactured, processed, packaged or held under contract by another company?				211.22
13. Have In-Process specifications been derived from process average and process variability estimates (validation)?				211.11
14. Is the individual responsible for Quality Assurance program not directly responsible for the performance of a manufacturing operation?				211.22
15. Are formal audits of the Quality Assurance program performed by individuals not having direct responsibility for the program?				211.180

	Response			Reference
	Yes	No	N/A	(21 CFR)
16. Are documented corrective actions taken on noted audit deficiencies?				211.180
17. Are the procedures for performing audits formalized?				211.180
18. Are the procedures available in an acceptable format for review by an FDA inspector?				211.180
19. Are production records retained at least one year beyond expiration date and two years beyond the date of release?				211.180

INTERNAL FACILITY AUDIT CHECKLIST

SECTION VII: PACKAGING, SHIPPING, AND DISTRIBUTION

	Response			Reference
	Yes	No	N/A	(21 CFR)
1. Is a check list used to verify shipping requirements?				211.20
2. Is product configuration verified prior to shipment?				211.150 211.196
3. Do packing and shipping records identify the individual performing and inspecting the shipping operation?				211.25
4. Are adequate storage facilities available and in use to safeguard the quality of the product between final acceptance and shipping?				211.42 211.142
5. Is there a distinct and adequate size label room?				211.42 211.122
6. Is the label room designed to avoid mix-ups?				211.42 211.122
7. Is there a sufficient accountability system for labels?				211.125
8. Are there specified restrictions on authority for access to labels and other labeling?				211.22(d)
9. Are labels proofread for accuracy before being released to inventory?				211.122

INTERNAL FACILITY AUDIT CHECKLIST

A: BIOPHARMACEUTICS

	Response			Reference
	Yes	No	N/A	(21 CFR)
1. Are the analytical lab facilities adequate to support its workload? Describe:				CP-Bio
2. Does the lab have written Standard Operating Procedures (SOPs)?				CP-Bio
3. Are the SOPs adequate, followed and available to personnel?				CP-Bio
4. Are analytical lab personnel capable of performing the required testing?				CP-Bio
5. Were CVs of analytical lab personnel available and reviewed?				CP-Bio

	Response			Reference
	Yes	No	N/A	(21 CFR)
6. Does the analytical lab receive blood or urine specimens for drug analysis? Describe: time and condition in prior clinic/ lab or in transit, etc.				CP-Bio
7. Were specimen storage conditions adequate before receipt at the analytical lab? Describe: special arrangements, shipping restriction, etc.				CP-Bio
8. Was dry ice used to ship specimens to the analytical lab?				CP-Bio
9. Will specimens be accepted at the analytical lab 24 hr/day, 7 days/wk? Describe special arrangements, shipping restrictions, etc.:				CP-Bio
10. Is a receipt log used to record the receiving of specimens, including conditions of samples, quantities, etc.?				CP-Bio
11. Was adequate equipment used to store specimens awaiting analysis? Describe:				CP-Bio
12. Does the above storage equipment have a warning device when not operating properly?				CP-Bio
13. Does the above storage equipment have a temperature recording device? Describe:				CP-Bio
14. Were the stored specimens in adequate condition? Describe: separation of samples, labels intact, broken, etc.				CP-Bio
15. Was the analytical equipment used adequate? Describe: models, conditions, etc.				CP-Bio
16. Were there written equipment operating procedures? Describe: adequate, available, etc.				CP-Bio
17. Were there written calibration/ standardization procedures for analytical equipment? Describe: adequate, used, frequency, etc.				CP-Bio
18. Are specific instrumental conditions recorded anywhere?				CP-Bio
19. For *Antibiotic Studies,* are incubators available? Describe: type, dimensions, etc.				CP-Bio
20. Are other conditions adequate? Describe: room temp. controlled, Petri dishes, zone readers, autoclaves, etc.				CP-Bio

	Response			Reference
	Yes	No	N/A	(21 CFR)
21. Is the analytical lab involved in the analysis of drug standards or products employed in a biopharmaceutic study? Describe: adequate, etc.				CP-Bio
22. For an *in vivo* analytical method, are there adequate data to document/validate claims on specificity, sensitivity, precision and stability?				CP-Bio
23. Did the analyst use coding techniques to blind samples?				CP-Bio
24. Was the order in which samples were analyzed adequate? Describe: randomized, in order, etc.				CP-Bio
25. Were test and reference samples run at the same time, under identical conditions?				CP-Bio
26. Were standard curves prepared for each batch of unknown samples? Describe: how often run, all reported, etc.				CP-Bio
27. Were blinded, spiked, control samples used in each CP-Bio run? Describe: who prepared, etc.				CP-Bio
28. Was the source of blank biological fluid adequate? Describe: use subject's zero hour sample, pooled plasma, etc.				CP-Bio
29. If samples were re-run, were control samples run simultaneously?				CP-Bio
30. Is there an adequate procedure defining whether an original or re-run value is reported?				CP-Bio
31. Are prepared reagents properly labeled? Describe: include chemist, storage condition, preparation date, expiration date, etc.				CP-Bio
32. For *Antibiotic Analyses*, were samples properly run through the incubator?				CP-Bio
33. Were control samples incubated at the same time, in the same incubator?				CP-Bio
34. Were other conditions adequate? Describe: temperature of incubator burner used to heat wire, zone readers used, etc.				CP-Bio
35. For *Radiometric Analyses* was the equipment used adequate? Describe: scintillation counter, etc.				CP-Bio

	Response			Reference
	Yes	No	N/A	(21 CFR)
36. Is the background level determined? How?				CP-Bio
37 Are bound notebooks used in the analytical lab?				CP-Bio
38. Are the procedures for filling in the notebooks adequate? Describe sequential entries, ink, chemist sign/date, how often, supervisor review/sign, etc.:				CP-Bio
39. Are all raw data (chromatograms, standard curves, etc.) retained? Describe: where chemist sign/date, supervisor review/ sign, etc.				CP-Bio
40. Are the procedures for maintenance of lab data adequate? Describe: "corrections," erasure, correction fluid, ink, record retention, etc.				CP-Bio

INTERNAL FACILITY AUDIT CHECKLIST

B: COMPUTER SYSTEMS VALIDATION

	Response			Reference
	Yes	No	N/A	(21 CFR)
1. Does the user feel that the computer system is comprised of hardware, software and a regulated application that warrants formal validation?				CS-Val
2. Does the interpretation of a "regulated application" include computerized data used in the assessment of safety or efficacy of a investigational drug?				CS-Val
3. Has the user identified/described the computer system to a Validation Board or management which agrees with the need for validation?				CS-Val
4. Is this computer system being purchased, in total or in part? Describe:				CS-Val
5. For an existing computer system, has it ever been validated before, in total or in part?				CS-Val

	Response			Reference
	Yes	No	N/A	(21 CFR)
6. Is this a new computer system just being developed?				CS-Val
7. Has an appropriate task force been identified to develop and validate this new system?				CS-Val
8. Was the system development life cycle approach used to develop the computer system?				CS-Val
9. Was a validation protocol developed up front to describe how the system would be validated?				CS-Val
10. Did the validation protocol identify all the necessary ingredients? Describe:				CS-Val
11. Does an adequate change control system exist? Describe: cover H/W, S/W, SOPs documented, etc.				CS-Val
12. Is the change control system based on change only? Describe: or also on time interval, whichever comes first?				CS-Val
13. Were test data sets used to test the modules/total system?				CS-Val
14. Did the test data sufficiently "stress" the system? Describe: extreme values, erroneous values, replications, etc.				CS-Val
15. If software is purchased, will the vendor give the user the program source code?				CS-Val
16. Is the vendor willing to "escrow" the source code with a third party?				CS-Val
17. Was training adequately addressed for the users of the system?				CS-Val
18. Was back-up for the system adequately addressed?				CS-Val
19. Are there adequate SOPs covering the necessary aspects of the system?				CS-Val
20. Are there formal approval of the system by the user and management?				CS-Val
21. Was a final validation package (documentation) prepared for the computer system?				CS-Val
22. Was the validation package approved by the Validation Board or management?				CS-Val
23. Will the Validation Board continue to monitor this system/changes in the future?				CS-Val

CHAPTER 8

MANAGING FDA INSPECTIONS

8.1 INTRODUCTION

When an FDA team visits a research, production, or other facility to conduct a scheduled or unscheduled investigation, many organizations react with barely controlled chaos. Plans are disrupted, anxieties surface, and otherwise calm and well-organized professional tremble. The result is likely to be added expense as casual investigator comments are taken as policy requirements; scheduled activities are delayed or disrupted; and carefully planned procedures are hastily revised.

International readers may find all of this confusing. Under the regulatory relationships operating in most countries, regulators frequently visit to help discuss new plans, to brainstorm ideas, and to facilitate new approaches. But the adversarial role of the FDA all too often makes visits major and traumatic events.

The costs associated with restructured procedures and delayed implementations can be minimized, however, with effective management of the FDA visit. Many regulatory professionals are not aware that they can control the FDA investigation to a large degree, and they passively respond rather than actively direct. But assuming an active role can help calm management and employees, can aid the FDA in their role, and can effectively contain the costs associated with this aspect of regulatory compliance.

Managing the visit process requires that the investigated organization have a Standard Operating Procedures for inspections in place, that staff be well-trained in how to respond to FDA questions and requests, that an effective regulatory professional be prepared to assume an active and directional role in the process, and that supporting documents be available and well-organized. These elements can be confirmed and honed by scheduling an independent or "mock" FDA audit prior to an anticipated visit. In fact, with the budgetary pressures facing the FDA, often the report of that mock visit, conducted by a credible and independent audit team, will supplement or supplant the FDA investigation. In many cases, the FDA will de facto accept the audit report in lieu of their own investigation.

Looking forward, as more and more organizations have independent audit reports available, and the FDA continues to face severe budgetary restraints, it is likely that the agency will evolve to the model used by the Securities and Exchange

Cost-Contained Regulatory Compliance: For the Pharmaceutical, Biologics, and Medical Device Industries, First Edition. Sandy Weinberg.
© 2011 John Wiley & Sons, Inc. Published 2011 by John Wiley & Sons, Inc.

Commission under which public companies are required to hire qualified and independent Certified Public Accountant firms to conduct regular audits. The SEC, in turn, reviews those reports and steps in directly only if a problem is suspected. This model, currently in use by ISO, CLIA, and a number of other organizations, represents a viable and high-expertise solution for allowing the FDA to effectively control a self-regulated process.

In the meantime, managing the FDA visit is the most effective strategy for minimizing costs associated with those on-site investigations.

8.2 CONFUSING PATHS

Before providing some effective and specific strategies for managing FDA inspections, visits, and investigations it is valuable to provide a simple matrix for understanding the sometimes confusing pathways that define these interactions. There are two primary dimensions that define the major types of FDA on site visits: crossing the two levels with two options each products a model with four possible strategic paths.

There are two general types of FDA on site experiences: "Routine" visits, in which a randomly scheduled visit is designed to confirm general compliance with GMP and other standards, are mandated to occur every two to three years, but in reality (as a result of budgetary limitations) are more likely to be scheduled on a five- to six-year cycle. "For Cause" inspections, on the other hand, are trigger by a specific problem, perhaps uncovered in a routine visit. "For cause" investigations may not be the result of any error or problem within a specific organization: The FDA may schedule a "For Cause" visit in response to a problem found with a specific class of drugs, or a processing methodology, or a specific segment of the industry.

Further complicating this dimension, the FDA has in place two distinct approaches to inspection. In the past three years the agency has introduced the concept of "Systems Inspections" to replace the older "Problem Inspection" approach. All field investigators have received at least basic training in the systems approach. However, reports from the industry suggest that in more than half of the recent visits, the investigators have ignored the system methodology to revert to the problem inspection approach.

It is possible, then, to have a Routine Systems visit; a Routine Problem visit, a For Cause Systems visit, or a For Cause Problem visit. While no reliable statistics are available, one can intuit that the most common investigations are Routine Systems and For Cause Problems.

In a Systems visit (either Routine or For Cause) an investigator begins by requesting a list of all of the systems in place in a specific site. This list might include Quality Assurance and Control, manufacturing, warehouse management, labeling and shipping, and so on. The QA/QC system is, of course, a critical feature of any GMP facility; other systems may vary significantly.

The investigator will then focus on the QA/QC system, and on one or more additional systems. In a For Cause investigation, the secondary systems selected will be related to the specific problem that triggered the visit. In a Random visit, the other systems are likely to be selected based upon an informal random process, upon the area of expertise of the specific investigator, upon a general area of concern observed at other recent visit to other companies, and upon any other factor.

In a Problem-oriented visit, the investigator will generally begin by requesting one or more specific Standard Operating Procedures. This review will then lead to a check for conformity to SOPs, and on to an examination of the controls and problem logs related to encountered procedures. Any observed problems trigger requests for additional documents, which in turn lead to checks for accuracy and conformity, additional problems, and so on. The path tends to be convoluted, and it complicates the managerial process.

Generally speaking, the Systems approach is most preferable for the company (and the agency), resulting a more carefully focused and organized visit. In addition, the Systems inspection has a major advantage: The visited organization knows in advance at least one of the areas of focus (QA/QC); an independent audit of that system can alleviate a great deal of the inspection pressure and can provide important reassurance to the visitation team.

8.3   ADVANCE PREPARATION

The key to successful management of an FDA visit, as in so much of life, is advance preparation. There are three specific actions that can be implemented to assist in controlling the FDA when on site: development of a formal Standard Operating Procedure (SOP) for visits; training of staff; and organization of documents.

The SOP for visits can direct the detailed actions of the FDA, but will only be considered valid if it applies uniformly to all site visitors; you cannot have one guideline for the FDA and another for client auditor, invited visitors, other regulatory agencies, or anyone else. But as long as the SOP is uniformly applied, is reasonable, and is provided at the beginning of the visit, most FDA investigators will make an effort to comply.

An effective SOP for Visitors might address such issues as:

- Prohibition against photography and sound recording
- Prohibition against unescorted wandering
- Requirement to identify affiliation before addressing any employee (i.e., "I'm and official with the FDA, and I'd like to ask ..." or "I'm a reporter with *Sixty Minutes*, can you tell me ...")
- Prohibition against removal of any original documents from the facility
- Requirement of conformity to all safety and security requirements
- Guidelines for appropriate gowning and gloving
- Requirement for a debriefing prior to departure

The final issue listed is particularly controversial and particularly important. It requires that visitors attend a debriefing meeting and provide feedback (verbally) on what they have observed or on any concerns they have developed. FDA investigators are generally hesitant to comply (no doubt to avoid contention and controversy), but a debriefing provides you with an opportunity to defuse any misunderstandings.

For example, a few years ago the author attended an FDA investigation of a pharmaceutical manufacturing site in Puerto Rico (where the native language is Spanish). At the beginning of the visit the FDA investigator requested access to all SOPs in use. The company guide looked confused, and he replied that they did not have any documents of that name. The visit would have ended with significant adverse findings had a debriefing not provided the company management with an opportunity to explain that they did have a complete set of POSs (the Spanish abbreviation for Standard Operating Procedures); what had seemed like a total disregard for GMP documentation requirements turned out to be a simple misunderstanding.

Similarly, prohibiting photographs and recordings can eliminate a significant source of intimidation on the part of staff members. In a legalistic society having an investigator record, your responses to questions is likely to prove frightening. If individuals are asked instead to initial the summaries of transcripts of their statements, they at least have an opportunity to correct or expand on comments.

These issues should be carefully considered, and a formal SOP for visits should be developed. A few "trial visits" from outside clients or independent auditors will quickly identify any additional issues. Once complete, the SOP should be formalized and posted (or made available) in the company lobby or visitors center.

Incidentally, Security or Reception personnel should be familiarized with the Visitor SOP, and they should be instructed to provide all visitors with access. They should also provide general notification to management and personnel that an FDA representative is on campus (some companies fly a specific flag from their flagpole). An FDA investigator expects to see your best performance—the conformity to guidelines and SOPS when you know they are watching.

One final note: Once an FDA investigator identifies him or herself (generally with a Federal Identification Card) a facility is required to grant admission with "all due speed"—generally interpreted as within an hour or so. The fact that the head of regulatory is off site, on vacation, or in a meeting isn't considered a viable excuse; there should be a plan in place to have alternate persons available.

8.4 TRAINING FOR FDA VISITS

FDA investigators are generally escorted by a designated member of the Regulatory Affairs department who is familiar with FDA policy, guidelines for inspections, and the visitation process. This designated escort will generally lead the team to an available conference room, review the SOP for Visitors with the FDA team, record the names and contact information of the team members (including Federal Identification numbers), and request the purpose of the visit.

At this first meeting the investigators will indicate whether the visit is routine or for cause, and whether or not it is a systems investigation. The escort may provide access to independent audit reports: these often provide the FDA investigators with all the information they require, and they may lead to a rapid and positive termination of the visit.

Assuming the visit moves forward, the FDA team may identify issues they are interested in, documents they wish to review, people they want to talk with, systems they want to inspect, or other concerns that may have prompted the visit. The escort will, of course, note these issues and will arrange access to requested documents, people, and locations. When documents that are missing controls are not in place, the escort should accurately report the deficiency; lying to a Federal official is a serious offense, and anything but clear and accurate responses are likely to significantly affect personal and corporate credibility, and to expand the scope of the visit.

These procedures are a standard part of the training and experience of any regulatory professional. But there are important regulatory principles that should be communicate to all organizational employees prior to any FDA visit. These principles should be a part of every employee's orientation training, should be reviewed regularly and perhaps posted prominently, and should be institutionalized as a part of the corporate culture.

8.5   TEN COMMANDMENTS FOR FDA VISITS

There are 10 basic rules for coping with FDA visits. Some companies post these commandments prominently for employee reference; some formalize them in a Standard Operating Procedure or Technical Operating Procedure. All organizations should probably incorporate them into employee training.

Importantly, these are not rules for tricking the FDA, or for circumventing regulations of inspections. In some military setting inspections are treated like a game, in which one side tries to hide problems while the other attempts to discover the deceptions. That attitude is not appropriate here, where everyone should share the goal of end user safety and health. The "commandments" described below have been developed with the assistance and concurrence of FDA field investigators: they are designed to smooth the process, not to hid rough areas.

1.   Answer All Questions Accurately

For legal, ethical, and reputational reasons, never attempt to falsify, deceive, or mislead. The consequences are series and potentially career ending (and may even result in criminal liability). Maintain a professional demeanor, and remember that the company and the FDA share a common goal of protecting patient health and safety.

2.   Agree on an Agenda

Request a clear statement on (a) the purpose of the visit and (b) the system or systems of interest. The scope of the visit may expand as observations are made, but a clear agenda should allow efficient use of everyone's time.

3. Answer Specific Questions

Don't volunteer information beyond the scope of the question, and don't run afield with your answers. A question phrased "Do you generally follow the procedure …?" isn't seeking a description of the exceptions; a question asking about problems encountered is inquiring about those that were found to be significant.

4. Follow the "Plan–Follow Through–Review" Formula

All actions should begin with a documented plan, and should conclude with a quality review to determine conformity to the plan goals. That formulation should be second nature, and it should be demonstrated for any significant activity. The appropriate answer (and appropriate process) for a question of "How did you …?" is generally "Here is the plan we developed in advance, here is the action we took, here is the analysis of the result."

5. Consider an SOP/TOP Construct

Some organizations have effectively experimented with a two-tier system of employee guidelines: (a) formalized, required Standard Operating Procedures and (b) less formal, more flexible Technical Operating Procedures. For example, an SOP may require that back-up copies of all data be stored in a secure, protected archive room. The TOP may specific which room or rooms are currently being utilized for that purpose. The advantage of the TOP is that major revisions and high-level approvals are not needed every time a new archive room is utilized.

If an SOP/TOP formulation is in use, inform the FDA visitors at first opportunity. The main criterion for acceptance is likely the clarity of directions to employees about what kinds of directions require SOP formality and which are appropriate for the more flexible TOPs.

If you are not using TOPs, make certain that all SOPs are up to date in the detail of actions they require. Should our SOP call for archive in room 109, add an appendix when space requirement forces you to begin using room 110.

6. Don't Brag, Complain, or Editorialize

An FDA visit is not the appropriate opportunity to air grievances about the agency, the government, the company, or supervisors. Do not attempt to use the visit as a "soapbox" to discuss peeves about policy or personnel.

7. Allow the Guide to Determine Who Should Respond

When the FDA visits, the company assigns a guide, generally the head of the Regulatory Department, to accompany all activities. If asked a question by the FDA visitor, give the Guide an opportunity to intervene if another employee if better suited to provide that response. The Guide may also clarify, or seek clarification, for the question.

8.   Note All Documents Requested

Whenever possible, provide photocopies (not originals) of documents requested. In any case, keep a log (or assist the Guide in doing so) or all documents provided to the FDA.

9.   Resolve Problems Promptly

If a problem is discovered, take immediate corrective action whenever appropriate. For example, in a recent visit an FDA represented noted that an SOP required that a storage room door remain closed; inspection showed that it had been temporarily propped open by an employee shifting files. The guide promptly closed the door, avoiding an adverse finding report.

10.   Request Debriefing

If you have a Visit SOP in place, it should require a debriefing; in any case, request that the FDA visitors verbally share their findings before departure. This is not an opportunity to debate, but it is a chance to clarify any misunderstandings and to begin immediate corrective action.

These 10 guidelines, or company appropriate policies of a similar nature, should form the backbone of employee FDA training and relations. While the order is arbitrary, care should be taken to emphasize the fundamental importance of the first commandment: Answer all questions accurately. Your organization's credibility is tantamount. If the FDA visitors appropriately believe that your company is devoted to high quality and compliance, everything else will fall in line: if they believe that your organization is trying to deceive, is cutting corners, or is not serious about quality, then the duration, depth, and cost of the visit will soar.

8.6   META CONSIDERATIONS

Using these 10 general guidelines, appropriate Good Manufacturing Practices training, and effective managerial leadership, there are three general meta principles to be internalized by all organizational employees. These meta considerations will lead to an effective and cost-contained relationship with the Food and Drug Administration: more importantly, they will assure the health and safety of the public as it relates to the organization's products.

First and most fundamental, complete honesty is a critical principle. There is no room for half-truths, exaggerations, evasions, or anything except the provision of full responses to all questions. The most important impression to make is of corporate credibility; that commodity is not worth risking for any short-term prize. If an FDA investigator is convinced that the organization shares the values of health and safety, much can be overlooked: if that investigator believes that the company is attempting to hide problems or disguise dangers, all problems become significant.

Second and closely related, it is important to build a positive relationship between the FDA and the organization. This relationship is not based on friendship but rather on common goals. The FDA is not primarily a regulatory agency; the regulatory role rests with the company and with its quality assurance/control and regulatory departments. The FDA's role is to assure the proper performance of the in-house regulatory team. Building a relationship of common concerns for product safety and for strict enforcement of standards and requirements will clearly establish this appropriate division of responsibilities. Build a relationship that says "we are concerned about quality even when you (the FDA) are not present."

Third, emphasize the importance of accuracy of detail. Inquiry responses should be met with specification, not generality. Consider the difference between responding to the question "How many rejects do you experience per thousand unit?" with "very few" versus "In our most recent study, conducted on October 3, we experienced a rejection rate of .03%, within the range experience in our three previous quarterly studies." The second response clearly shows organization, control, and self-reliant internal regulation.

Those three characteristics—organization, control, and self-regulation—are the primary determinant goals of an FDA visit. Your goals are to demonstrate that your organization is effectively organized, able to identify and supply planning documents, reports, and inventories in a timely manner. You should be able to (a) point to an appropriate system of Standard Operating Procedures that demonstrate control of operations and (b) prove that those SOPs are carefully followed throughout the organization. And your company must demonstrate that you self-regulate—that is, that your quality assurance and control unit provides daily oversight of the same fundamental principles guidelines and regulations that the FDA can only spot check.

When that organization, control, and self-regulation are demonstrated in an honest, credible, accurate manner, FDA visits will be effectively cost-controlled, without the added expensive burden of product recalls, approval delays, and loss of credibility.

APPENDIX TO CHAPTER 8

Here are two tools to assist in self-regulation: a GLP Compliance Facility Inspection Checklist, keyed to appropriate FDA requirements (appropriate for laboratory and research environments), and the equivalent GLP Checklist, appropriate for manufacturing and other environments.

GLP COMPLIANCE FACILITY INSPECTION

21 CFR PART 58

TOPIC	YES	NO	N/A	COMMENTS
A. General Provisions 58.10				
1. Has the sponsor in utilizing the services of a consulting laboratory, contractor, or grantee to perform an analysis or other service notified them that the service is part of a nonclinical laboratory study and must be conducted in compliance with the provisions of this part?				
B. Personnel 58.29				
1. Does each individual engaged in the conduct of or supervision of the study have the education, training and experience to perform the assignments?				
2. Does the facility maintain a current summary of training, experience and job descriptions for each person engaged in or supervising the study?				
3. Are there sufficient personnel for the timely and proper conduct of the study according to the protocol?				

(Continued)

Cost-Contained Regulatory Compliance: For the Pharmaceutical, Biologics, and Medical Device Industries, First Edition. Sandy Weinberg.
© 2011 John Wiley & Sons, Inc. Published 2011 by John Wiley & Sons, Inc.

TOPIC	YES	NO	N/A	COMMENTS
4. Does personnel take sanitation and health precautions to avoid contamination of test and control articles and test systems?				
5. Does personnel engage in the study, wear appropriate clothing, and changed at a frequency to prevent microbiological, radiological, or chemical contamination of test systems and test and control articles?				
6. Are personnel with an illness that may adversely affect the test systems, test and control articles and any other operation excluded form the study until corrected?				
7. Is personnel instructed to report to their super any health or medical conditions that may have an adverse effect on the study?				
C. Testing Facility Management 58.31				
1. Does the testing facility management:				
• Designate a Study Director before study initiation?				
• If necessary, replace the Study Director promptly?				
• Document and maintain replacement of the Study Director as raw data?				
• Assure there is a Quality Assurance Unit (QAU) established?				
• Assure that test and control articles or mixtures are appropriately tested for identity, strength, purity, stability and uniformity, as applicable?				
• Assure that personnel, resources, facilities, equipment, materials, and methodologies are available as scheduled?				
• Assure that personnel clearly understand the functions they are to perform?				
• Assure that any deviations from these regulations reported by the QAU are communicated to the Study Director and corrective actions are taken and documented?				

TOPIC	YES	NO	N/A	COMMENTS
D. Study Director 58.33				
1. Does the Study Director have appropriate education, training and experience?				
2. Does the Study Director exercise overall responsibility for the technical conduct of the study, including interpretation, analysis, documentation, and reporting of results?				
3. Does the Study Director assure:				
• That the protocol and changes are approved as provided by 58.120 and followed?				
• That all experimental data, including observations of unanticipated responses to the test system are accurately recorded and verified?				
• That unforeseen circumstances that may affect the quality and integrity of the study are noted when they occur and corrective action is taken and documented?				
• That test systems are as specified in the protocol?				
• That all applicable good laboratory practice regulations are followed?				
• That all raw data, documentation, protocols, specimens and final reports are transferred to the archives during or at the close of the study?				
E. Quality Assurance Unit 58.35				
1. Consist of one or more individuals responsible for monitoring.				
2. Assures management facilities, equipment, personnel, methods, records, etc., in conformance.				
3. Separate, independent of those directing, conducting.				
4. Maintain copy of master schedule as required.				
5. Maintain copies of relevant protocols.				

(Continued)

TOPIC	YES	NO	N/A	COMMENTS
6. Periodically inspect each phase and document.				
7. Immediately inform Study Director of significant problems likely to affect integrity.				
8. Periodically submit to management and Study Director reports, including corrective actions.				
9. No deviation from protocols of SOPs made without authorization and documentation.				
10. Review final report assuring it is accurate andreflects raw data.				
11. Issue QAU statement for inclusion in finalreport.				
12. SOPs of responsibilities, procedures, records,maintained, method of indexing.				
13. Maintain record with inspection dates, study,phase, inspector.				
14. Assure inspections done according to GLP.				
F. Facilities 58.41				
1. Suitable size, construction, location for properconduct.				
2. Provides separation preventing adverse effect.				
G. Animal Care Facilities 58.43				
1. Does the facility have a sufficient number of animal rooms or areas as needed, to assure proper:				
• Separation of species or test systems?				
• Isolation of individual projects?				
• Quarantine of animals?				
• Routine or specialized housing of animals?				
2. Does the facility have a number of rooms separate from those above to ensure isolation of studies being done with test systems or test and control articles known to be biohazardous including materials and infectious agents?				
3. Are separate areas provided for the diagnosis, treatment, and control of laboratory animal diseases?				

TOPIC	YES	NO	N/A	COMMENTS
4. Do these areas provide effective isolation for the housing animals either known or suspected of being diseased or of being carriers of disease form other animals?				
5. Do the facilities provide for the collection and disposal of all animal waste and refuse or for safe sanitary storage of waste before removal from the facility?				
6. Are the disposal facilities provided and operated as to minimize vermin infestation, odors, disease hazards and environmental contamination?				
7. Are the facilities designed, constructed and located so as to minimize disturbances that interfere with the study?				
H. Animal Supply Facilities 58.45				
1. Are there storage areas, as needed, for feed, bedding, supplies and equipment?				
2. Are the storage areas for feed and bedding separated from areas housing the test systems?				
3. Are these storage areas protected against infestation or contamination?				
I. Facilities for Handling Test and Control Articles 58.47				
1. As necessary to prevent contamination mix-ups, are there separate areas for:				
• Receipt and storage of the test and control articles?				
• Mixing of the test and control articles with a carrier, e.g. feed?				
• Storage of the test and control article mixtures?				
2. Are storage areas for the test and/or control article and test and control mixtures separate from areas housing the test systems?				
3. Are they adequate to preserve the identity, strength, purity, and stability of the articles and mixtures?				

(Continued)

TOPIC	YES	NO	N/A	COMMENTS
J. Laboratory Operation Areas 58.49				
1. Is separate laboratory space provided for the performance of the routine procedures including specialized areas for performing activities such as aseptic surgery, intensive care, necropsy, histology, radiography, and handling of biohazardous materials?				
2. Is separate space provided for cleaning, sterilizing, and maintaining equipment and supplies used during the course of the study?				
K. Specimen and Data Storage Facilities 58.51				
1. Is space provided for archives, limited to access by authorized personnel only, for the storage and retrieval of all raw data and specimens from completed studies?				
L. Equipment Design 58.61				
1. Is the automatic, mechanical or electronic equipment used in the generation, measurement or assessment of data and equipment used for facility environmental control or appropriate design and adequate capacity to function according to the protocol?				
2. Is this equipment suitably located for operation, inspection, cleaning, and maintenance?				
M. Maintenance and Calibration of Equipment 58.63				
1. Is this equipment adequately inspected, cleaned and maintained?				
2. Is equipment used for the generation, measurement or assessment of data adequately tested, calibrated, and/or standardized?				
3. Do the standard operating procedures (SOP) required in 58.81 (b)(11) set forth in sufficient detail the methods, materials, and schedules to be used in the routine inspection, cleaning, maintenance, testing, calibration, and/or standardization of equipment?				

TOPIC	YES	NO	N/A	COMMENTS
4. Do these SOPs specify the remedial action to be taken in the event of failure or malfunction of equipment?				
5. Do these SOPs also designate the person responsible for the performances of each operation?				
6. Are copies of the SOPs made available to laboratory personnel?				
7. Are written records maintained of all inspection, maintenance, testing, calibration, and/or standardizing operations?				
8. Do these records, containing the date of operation, describe whether the maintenance operations were routine and followed the written SOPs?				
9. Are written records kept of nonroutine repairs performed on equipment as a result of failure and malfunction?				
10. Do these records document the nature of the defect, how and when the defect was discovered, and any remedial action taken in response to the defect?				
N. Standard Operating Procedures 58.81				
1. SOPs written to ensure data quality, integrity.				
2. Changes in SOPs authorized.				
3. SOPs established, but not limited to:				
• Animal room preparation.				
• Animal care.				
• Receipt, identification, storage, handling, mixing and method of sampling TCA.				
• Test systems observations.				
• Laboratory tests.				
• Handling of animals found moribund or dead.				

(Continued)

TOPIC	YES	NO	N/A	COMMENTS
• Necropsy or postmortem examinations.				
• Collection and identification of specimens.				
• Histopathology.				
• Data handling, storage and retrieval.				
• Maintenance and calibration of equipment.				
• Transfer, placement and identification of animals.				
4. Relevant SOPs, manuals immediately available.				
5. Literature supplement to SOPs not in lieu of.				
6. Historical file of SOPs and all revisions.				
7. Computer SOPs for:				
• Software/computer program validation.				
• Maintenance of computer equipment.				
• Approval of Software changes.				
• Security of the computer system.				
• Computer "downtime".				
O. Reagents and Solutions 58.83				
1. Are all reagents and solutions in the laboratory areas labeled to indicate identity, titer or concentrations, storage requirements, and expiration date?				
2. Are deteriorated or outdated reagents and solutions not used?				
P. Animal Care 58.90				
1. Is there a SOP for housing, feeding, handling, and care of animals?				
2. Are all newly received animals from outside sources placed in quarantine until their health status has been evaluated?				
3. Are these evaluations in accordance with acceptable veterinary medical practice?				

TOPIC	YES	NO	N/A	COMMENTS
4. At the initiation of the study are the animals free of any disease or condition that might interfere with the purpose or conduct of the study?				
5. In the course of a study are the animals that contract such a disease or condition isolated?				
6. If these animals are treated for the disease or signs of the disease does the treatment not interfere with the study?				
7. Are the diagnosis, authorizations of treatment, and each date of treatment documented and retained?				
8. Do warm-blooded animals, excluding suckling rodents, used in laboratory procedures that require manipulations and observations over an extended period of time receive appropriate identification (e.g., tattoo, toe clip, color code, ear tag, ear punch, etc.)?				
9. Do these above type animals used in studies that require the animals to be removed from and returned to their home cages for any reason (e.g., cage cleaning, treatment, etc.)?				
10. Does all information needed to specifically identify each animal within an animal-housing unit appear on the outside of that unit?				
11. Are animals of different species housed in separate rooms when necessary?				
12. Are animals of the same species, but used in different studies, not ordinarily housed in the same room when inadvertent exposure to control or test articles or animal mix-up which could affect the outcome of either study?				
13. If such mixed housing is necessary, is adequate differentiation by space and identification made?				
14. Are animal cages, racks, and accessory equipment cleaned and sanitized at appropriate intervals?				

(Continued)

TOPIC	YES	NO	N/A	COMMENTS
15. Are feed and water used for the animals analyzed periodically to ensure that contaminants known to be capable of interfering with the study and reasonably expected to be present in such feed or water not present at levels above those specified in the protocol?				
16. Are such analyses maintained as raw data?				
17. Does the bedding used in animal cages or pens interfere with the purpose or conduct of the study?				
18. Is the bedding changed as often as necessary to keep the animals dry and clean?				
19. If pest control materials are used, is their use documented?				
20. Are cleaning and pest control materials that interfere with the study not used?				
Q. Test and Control Article Characterization 58.105				
1. The identity, strength, purity, and composition or other characteristics that will appropriately define the test or control article determined and documented for each batch?				
2. Are the methods of synthesis, fabrication or derivation of the test and control articles documented by the sponsor or the testing facility?				
3. Are marketed products used as control articles characterized by their labeling?				
4. Is the stability of each test or control article determined by the testing facility or by the sponsor before initiation of a study or concomitantly according to SOP, which provides for periodic reanalysis of each batch?				
5. Is each storage container for a test or control article labeled by name, chemical abstract number or code number, batch number, expiration date, if any and where appropriate, storage conditions necessary to maintain the identity, strength purity, and composition of the test or control article?				

TOPIC	YES	NO	N/A	COMMENTS
6. Are storage containers assigned to a particular test article of the duration of the study?				
7. For studies lasting more than 4 weeks' duration, are reserve samples from each batch of test and control articles retained for the period of time provided in 58.195?				
R. Test and Control Article Handling 58.107				
1. Are procedures established for a system for handling of the test and control articles to ensure that:				
• There is proper storage?				
• Distribution is made in a manner designed to preclude the possibility of contamination, deterioration or damage?				
• Proper identification is maintained throughout the distribution process?				
• The receipt and distribution of each batch is documented, including the date and quantity of each batch distributed or returned?				
S. Mixtures of Articles with Carriers 58.113				
1. For each test or control article that is mixed with a carrier, are tests by appropriate analytical methods conducted:				
• To determine that uniformity of the mixture and to determine, periodically, the concentration of the test or control article in the mixture?				
• To determine the stability of the test and control articles in the mixture?				
2. If the stability cannot be determined before initiation of the study, are SOPs established and followed to provide for periodic re-analysis of the test and control articles in the mixtures?				
3. Do any of the components of the test and control article carrier mixture have an expiration date, and is that date clearly shown on the container?				

(Continued)

TOPIC	YES	NO	N/A	COMMENTS
4. If more than one component has an expiration date, is the earliest date shown?				
T. Protocol for and Conduct of a Nonclinical Laboratory Study 58.120				
1. Does each study have an approved written protocol that clearly indicates the objectives and all methods for the conduct of the study?				
2. Does the protocol contain, but is not necessarily limited to, the following information:				
• A descriptive title and statement of the purpose of the study?				
• Identification of the test and control articles by name, chemical, abstract number or code number?				
• The name of the sponsor and the name and address of the testing facility at which the study is being conducted?				
• The proposed starting and completion dates?				
• Justification for selection of the test system?				
• A description of the experimental design, including the methods for control of bias?				
• A description and/or identification of diet used in the study as well as solvent, emulsifiers, and/or materials used to solubilize or suspend the test or control articles before mixing with the carrier?				
• A description including specifications for acceptable levels of contaminants that are reasonably expected to be present in the dietary materials and are known to be capable of interfering with the purpose or conduct of the study if present at levels greater than established by the specifications?				
• The route of administration?				
• The reason for route of administration choice?				

TOPIC	YES	NO	N/A	COMMENTS
• Each dosage level, expressed in milligrams per kilogram of body weight or other appropriate units, of the test or control article to be administered and the method article to be administered and the method and frequency of administration?				
• Method by which the degree of absorption of the test and control articles by the test system will be determined if necessary to achieve the objectives of study?				
• The type and frequency of test, analyses and measurements to be made?				
• The records to be maintained?				
• The date of approval of the protocol by the sponsor and the signature of the Study Director?				
• A statement of the proposed statistical methods to be used?				
3. Are all the changes in or revisions of an approved protocol and the reasons documented, signed by the Study Director, dated and maintained with the protocol?				
U. Conduct of a Nonclinical Laboratory Study 58.130				
1. Data recorded directly, promptly, legibly, ink.				
2. Entry dated on day of entry, signed by same person.				
3. Changes do not obscure, give reason, dated and signed at time of change.				
4. Individual responsible direct computer input identified at time of data input.				
5. Changes in computer entries do not obscure, given reason, dated identify responsible individual.				

(Continued)

TOPIC	YES	NO	N/A	COMMENTS
V. Storage and Retrieval of Records and Data 58.190				
1. Are all raw data, documentation, protocols, specimens, and final reports generated as a result of a nonclinical laboratory study retained?				
2. Is there an archives for orderly storage and expedient retrieval of all raw data, documentation, protocols, specimens, and interim and final reports?				
3. Do the conditions of storage minimize deterioration of the documents or specimens in accordance with the requirements for the time period of their retention and the nature of the documents or specimens?				
4. If the facility has contracted with a commercial archive to provide a repository for all material to be retained, has specific reference been made in the archive to those other locations?				
5. Is an individual identified as responsible for the archives?				
6. Do only authorized personnel enter the archive?				
7. Is material retained or referred to in the archives indexed by test article, date of study, test system, and nature of study?				
W. Retention of Records 58.195				
1. Except for wet specimens, samples of test or control articles, and specially prepared material (e.g. histochemical, electron microscopic, blood mounts, teratological preparation and uteri from dominant lethal mutagenesis tests), are documentation records, raw data and specimens pertaining to a non-clinical laboratory study and required to be made by this part retained in the archive(s) for whichever of the following periods is shortest:				
• A period of at least 2 years following the date on which an application for a research or marketing permit, in support of which the results of the nonclinical laboratory study were submitted, is approved by the FDA?				

TOPIC	YES	NO	N/A	COMMENTS
• A period of at least 5 years following the date on which the results of the nonclinical laboratory study are submitted to the FDA in support of an application for a research or marketing permit?				
• In other situations (e.g., where the nonclinical laboratory study does not result in the submission of the study in support of an application for a research or marketing permit), a period of at least 2 years following date on which the study is completed, terminated or discontinued?				
2. Are wet specimens, samples of test or control articles, and specially prepared material (e.g. histochemical, electron microscopic, blood mounts, teratological preparation and uteri from dominant lethal mutagenesis tests) retained only as long as the quality of the preparation affords evaluation?				
3. Are the master schedule sheet, copies of protocols, and records of quality assurance inspections, as required by 58.35 maintained by the quality assurance unit as an easily accessible system of records for the period of time specified in 1 and 2 of this section?				
4. Are summaries of training and experience and job descriptions required to be maintained by 58.29 retained along with all other testing facility employment records for the length of time specified in 1 and 2 of this section?				
5. Are records and reports of the maintenance and calibration and inspection of equipment, as required by 58.63, retained for the length of time specified in (2) of this section?				
6. If a facility conducting nonclinical testing goes out of business, are all raw data, documentation, and other material specified in this section transferred to the archives of the sponsor of the study?				
7. If the above transfer occurs is the FDA notified in writing?				

(Continued)

GUIDELINE FOR DOCUMENTATION IN THE GLP VACCINE LABORATORY

1.0 INTRODUCTION

The transition from an academic or basic research laboratory environment to a facility in compliance with the Food and Drug Administration's Good Laboratory Practices (GLPs) involves a number of refocusing activities. Perhaps most challenging among them is the attitude adjustment required regarding documentation. In the FDA world documentation is the primary evidence of any activity: In regulatory parlance, if it wasn't documented, it wasn't done.

1.1 *Importance of documentation:* While this emphasis on documentation is largely related to the training, orientation and background of field investigators (evaluating documents is easier than evaluating activities), its premiere importance is nevertheless real. And a well-documented laboratory has three important advantages:

    1.1.1 *Regulatory:* As suggested above, it is easier to regulate a well-documented environment than to regulate a well-documented activity. As a self-regulated industry, using internal Quality Assurance units as the primary review unit (with the FDA serving as backup and watchdog), effective documentation provides a structure to the monitoring process.

    1.1.2 *Trace:* An important part of that regulatory process involves the ability to trace a final product back to its production and research roots and to trace a research direction or culture forward to its ultimate clinical destination. This trace is important in the event of a future problem, contamination, side effect, or adverse reaction.

    1.1.3 *Reference:* The essence of science is repeatability. Effective documentation of an experiment, process, result, procedure, or examination provides the pathway necessary to review and repeat. Without documentation the repeated experiment might be modified in some undetermined but critical dimension.

1.2 *Key Issues:* All documents must meet certain key criteria if the documents are to prove useful. In effect, these criteria represent an operating definition of an effective document.

    1.2.1 *Accurate:* The document must accurately describe the event, procedure, result, conclusion, output, observation, or process. Deviations from accuracy throw the entire document under a cloud of suspicion and renders its value moot.

    1.2.2 *Clear:* Ambiguous, incomplete, or unclear statements of process, analysis, procedure, or conclusion lead to confusion and misinterpretation. At the same time, it is important that a document not add inappropriate clarity to obtained results that are murky or ambiguous. As contradictory as it may sound, an effective document should be clear, including clearly stating any observed ambiguity.

    1.2.3 *Comprehensive:* Effective documentation must be comprehensive, including all relevant steps, data, and observations. Changes in contents should be tracked (presumably with an audit trail for data).

    1.2.4 *Current:* Documents should be dated and version controlled to assure that they represent current or time fixed situations.

1.2.5 *Available:* While offsite archives are acceptable and often desirable, there should be an effective method of locating and recalling documents. "Live" documents should be retained on site at the point of use for ready reference.

1.3 *Format:* The specific format of documents will vary, of course, according to the type of document. However, there are some general formatting criteria.

    1.3.1 *Pagination:* In written (non-electronic) documents, affirmative evidence that the document is complete is critical.

        1.3.1.1 No missing pages: Any intentional blank pages should be so marked ("Intentionally left blank" or equivalent). To prove completeness, a bound book, number/total paging ("page one of seven"), or other indication that no page has been deleted should be used.

        1.3.1.2 Index: Documents should include a table of contents, index, or equivalent inventory of contents.

    1.3.2 *Approvals:* All completed documents should have attached an approval page (or equivalent), with appropriate signatures and dates of approval. In some situations, approvals may include the recording scientists or author, a representative of Quality Assurance, and a representative of organizational management.

    1.3.3 *Consistent:* All documents within a given category (data, Standard Operating Procedures, etc.) should follow a consistent format for ease of analysis. That format should include a versioning system to assure that duplicates are accurate copies with a recall and replacement procedure. Past versions should be retained in a historical record.

1.4 *Archiving:* An archive of all historical records and "live" documents should be maintained. The key issues in archiving are preservation and retrieval.

    1.4.1 *Preservation:* Paper, film, microfiche, cultures, tissues, magnetic, and laser disk documents should be stored in a location providing protection from potentially destructive elements (heat, water, magnetic interference, etc.). In the case of paper and electronic data, only true copies (non-originals) should be permitted removal from the archive.

    1.4.2 *Retrieve:* Effective retrieval requires indexing. Generally, a document or equivalent should be capable of recall within forty-eight hours of request. Documents should be retained indefinitely.[1]

2.0 STANDARD OPERATING PROCEDURES (SOPS)

2.1 *Concept:* Standard Operating Procedures (SOPs) are the fundamental control documents in any vaccine laboratory. They describe how to conduct studies, record results, calibrate equipment, etc.

    2.1.1 *Management Control:* An SOP is considered to be the appropriate procedure to follow as determined and defined by the laboratory management.

---

[1] The FDA has provided guidelines for retention, varying by circumstance between three and ten years. However, the US Federal Courts have not recognized these guidelines and have in the past ruled that the inability to produce documents, regardless of FDA retention requirements, substantially weaken claims of testing and control.

That is, an alternate procedure, while intrinsically equivalent or superior, is considered an unacceptable violation of Standard Operating Procedures. The SOP not only dictates activities; it represents management control of those activities.

2.1.2 *Competent Professional:* An SOP need not be written for a naïve worker if the laboratory utilizes competent and trained professionals. For example, one could direct a lab worker to perform a chromatography test without specifying all of the preparatory and procedural steps in that test as long as the training or education of the workers is on file.

2.1.3 *Approved Procedures:* SOPs should be available to workers at the point of procedure for refresher reference as needed. In addition, SOPs may be used as training tools in orienting a worker to the procedure in question. Because these dual functions (reference and training) often result in multiple copies, it is critically important that a versioning and replacement/recall process be in place to be certain that all copies of a given SOP are identical. Photocopies should be prohibited, controlled, or restricted. While electronic SOPs may seem to solve this issue, special care must be made if workers are permitted to print copies of electronic SOPs.

2.1.4 *Technical Operating Procedures:* Some organization incorporate outside documents within SOPs. For example, an SOP for equipment use may refer workers to a user manual or instruction manual. These secondary documents are collectively identified as "Technical Operating Procedures" (TOPs). As long as they are controlled by policies stated in the SOP, TOPs are appropriate training materials, references, and more detailed guides.

2.2 *Approval Process:* SOPs generally require approval by a:

2.2.1 *Responsible Person:* This would be management.

2.2.2 *Quality Assurance Personal:* QA would check for accuracy, completeness, conformity to format, etc.

2.2.3 *Corporate Officer:* Who would acknowledge responsibility.

A date and the title of the signor should accompany all signatures.

2.3 *Content:* Standard Operating Procedures are expected to be directives, providing clear and unambiguous steps to be followed in accomplishing a given task. In effect, the SOP represents an operational definition of a procedure. For example, the goal of a hypothetical experiment might be to determine whether or not volunteer subjects are "tall." The SOP might operationalize that concept by directing that height be recorded in centimeters with subjects standing barefooted with their spine against a wall, taking three separate measurements at crown of skull and averaging the results.

Care should be taken to avoid:

2.3.1 *Undefined Options:* If multiple pathways are acceptable, there should be clear criteria for selecting between them.

2.3.2 *Ambiguous Activities:* Often having an outside reader review directions helps to identify hidden assumptions or ambiguities.

2.3.3 *Unnecessary Vague or Overly Specific Directions:* If a specific volume flask is required, it should be so identified. However, directing the worker to remove the flask from "the third shelf on the left" may cause confusion if flasks are relocated.

2.3.4 *Use of Names:* Persons to perform activities should be defined by job responsibility or title to avoid confusion in absence or reassignment.

2.4 *Electronic Standard Operating Procedures:* The regulation 21 CFR Part 11, "Electronic Signatures and Records," provides for the optional use of electronic documents, including SOPs. Part 11 requires that electronically signed documents (such as SOPs) meet three tests:

2.4.1 *Unique Identifier:* Through a dedicated password system biometric or other methodology the individual signing the document is clearly and uniquely identified.

2.4.2 *Locked Document:* The act of signing the document requires an affirmative action and serves to lock out any changes in the document subsequent to the signing.

2.4.3 *Time/Date Stamp:* When the document is affirmatively signed, a time/date stamp, indicating the time zone, location, or alternate identifier of sequence, is affixed.

Electronic SOPs carry the significant advantages of easy accessibility (presumably from any computer terminal) and of easy control of revisions (previous electronic versions are instantly replaced throughout the system).

Balanced against these advantages are two disadvantages, one significant and one minor. Significantly, if the system is nonfunctional, making the SOPs inaccessible, the activity controlled by the SOPs must be halted. Reliance on a paper back-up copy de facto defines the paper copy as the "real" SOP, and requires a manual revision system. Of less common occurrence, certain physical environments may preclude computer use (some warehouses, for example), making a paper system necessary.

2.5 *Standard Operating Procedures for a Laboratory:* The following topics should be included in SOPs:

2.5.1 Maintenance

2.5.2 Security

2.5.3 Quality Assurance

2.5.4 Laboratory Testing

2.5.5 Equipment Qualification

2.5.6 Records and Archiving

2.5.7 Laboratory Safety

2.5.8 Use and Training

2.5.9 Software Validation

3.0 DATA

Most laboratories input samples and output data for analysis and interpretation. That data are recorded as some form of documentation, paper, electronic, slides, tissues, or other biological artifacts. FDA requirements call for retaining the raw data to allow future reanalysis (the retention period is not clearly defined and has been effectively trumped by the Federal courts).

3.1 *Raw Data Defined:* The FDA has never provided a clear and consistent definition of "raw data," but other agencies,[2] whose definitions prevail in the absence of a specific FDA definition, have provided a weak but useable operationalization.

A laboratory *(or other regulated entity)* may define as "raw data" any archive from the collection path that precedes modification, classification or interpretation. That is, a scientist collecting tumor cells might classify as "raw" and retain the cells themselves, the output of the analytical device that describes (but does not interpret) those cells; the database that reports the device output; a photocopy of that database; et cetera. Once the results are analyzed, however, the data is no longer considered "raw" and must be retained prior to that point.

In practicality, most laboratories retain all stages of data (the tumor, the descriptive instrument output, the database, etc.). The general guideline is that, at some future date, it should be possible to repeat the analysis of the data.

Inherent in this situation are two sub-issues:

3.1.1 *Pre-define:* The laboratory must document a clear situational definition prior to the analysis (i.e., decide in advance to retain tumor cells or whatever as raw data).

3.1.2 *Consistent:* The definition utilized must be consistent for a specific application (i.e., retain all tumor cells in the study).

3.2 *Recording:* Paper or electronic data must be recorded.

3.2.1 *Manual:* Data should be recorded in a designated bound notebook in ink.

3.2.1.1 Any corrections or changes should be explained with rationale, data and signature of recorder.

3.2.1.2 There must be a clear indication that no pages have been deleted or removed from the laboratory notebook.

3.2.2 *Electronic:* Electronic data may be entered into a database directly from analytical or descriptive equipment or manually by a trained laboratory worker.

3.2.2.1 Audit trail: There must be an electronic[3] audit trail tracking any changes in the raw data file and indicating the reason, approving person, and time/date.

3.2.3 *Approval:* All data files (electronic and manual) should be signed and dated, identifying the time they were created and the person responsible for the creation. Some laboratories affix a QA signature to the original file; others conduct a QA review subsequent to the file creation.

3.3 *Archive:* As specified above, the raw data should be arrived in a manner and location that assures preservation, access, and ready retrieval.

4.0 SUPPORTING DOCUMENTATION

Most laboratories generate and collect a variety of supporting documentation. This includes the results of in-house and third party audits, documents related to the laboratory design

---

[2] Most specifically, the Environmental Protection Agency in its "Good Automated Laboratory Practices".

[3] During the transition period to Part 11 the FDA has accepted a carefully controlled manual audit trail—in effect, an accompanying laboratory notebook recording changes, as a temporary method.

and equipment installation, EEO and OSHA postings, et cetera. These documents should be available for review[4] or posted as appropriate.

These supplemental documents are subject to the following controls:

4.1   *Accessible Archive:* supplemental documents should be archived according to the standards applying to other forms of documentation, including preservation, retention, and recall.

4.2   *Review:* supplemental documents should be reviewed by appropriate management, Quality Assurance, and laboratory personnel. Some organizations require that reviewers initial and date their review, though this is not a universal requirement.

5.0   SUMMARY

The documentation of activities, data, and analytical results is a standard part of any scientific laboratory, formalized and magnified in a GLP regulatory situation. In general, all aspects of the operation should be documented, reviewed, signed and data, and retained in a secure archive.

Laboratories converting from research and development to GLP regulatory environments will generally need to add documented Standard Operating Procedures to govern all aspects of operations (including the generation, review, and archiving of documentation). These SOPs provide the skeletal structure that leads to the creation of effective documentary evidence of all aspects in the laboratory environment.

---

[4] Draft documents and works-in-progress are not intended for review by regulatory inspectors.

CHAPTER 9

RISK ASSESSMENT

9.1 INTRODUCTION

While the concept of Risk was touched on in the previous discussion of Quality by Design, the topic pervades all aspects of regulatory compliance and represents an effective cost-containment strategy in its own right. In fact, the regulatory concept of risk assessment was born in an effort to control regulatory costs.

All pharmaceutical, biologics, and device regulatory agencies—international historical, and global—are handicapped by a set of internally contradictory goals. The agency must devise strategies for securing the safety of the products they regulate, assuring that the protection of the public the agency is designed to protect. But at the same time, this regulatory agency must provide for appropriate access to those products, assuring the public of timely and needed therapies, preventatives, and treatments. If the scale tips too far toward safety, the constituency is deprived of needed therapeutics; if the access is too generous, unsafe products may be distributed. All regulatory agencies agonize over the ideal balance: The FDA has historically maximized safety at the loss of access. As a result, for example, the United States has the world's smallest, and arguably the most safe, pharmacopeia.

As the United States faced an increasing health cost crisis in the early years of the twenty-first century, the FDA and the industry began to reach consensus that regulation which did not increase public safety but which did add to the expense of producing pharmaceutical biologics, and device products effectively economically decreased public access to these products. Affordability became an issue, and strategies for minimizing expense without decreasing safety became critical.

Risk analysis represents such a strategy. It effectively offers a reliable method of determining where to and where not to apply regulatory guidelines, presumably decreasing cost (and increasing access) where safety issues are not significant.

9.2 RISK ASSESSMENT

The diverse and complex FDA guidelines, regulations, rules, and intiatives can be traced back to three foundation concepts that underlie all of the agency's philosophy. Those three principles can be used heuristically as well, providing a basis for

Cost-Contained Regulatory Compliance: For the Pharmaceutical, Biologics, and Medical Device Industries, First Edition. Sandy Weinberg.
© 2011 John Wiley & Sons, Inc. Published 2011 by John Wiley & Sons, Inc.

prediction of future FDA actions and a projection of interpretations and emphases. Since the FDA inception, these three principles have governed the ebb and flow of debate between proponents of the industry-promotion and protection (providing more medical options) versus public health and safety (providing fewer but safer options).

The first of these trends is that of **proximal causality**. Consider what may be the most basic of FDA regulatory models: A consumer purchases a simple medical device—perhaps a bandage—in a sterile container. That consumer has a right to expect that the package contains a sterile gauze pad. Public health and consumer confidence are maintained as long as the label is accurate and the final product is clean.

But is it enough that the final bandage contains no rat feces or beetle parts? Does the consumer have a right to be certain that those unhealthy extraneous ingredients were not simply sifted out just prior to radiation and to packing? Most consumers would respond affirmatively, and so regulators are authorized to investigate the packing plant itself to be certain that it is free of infestation.

And if that packing plant processes raw materials to eliminate those contaminants, should regulators also focus on the cleanliness and operation of that processing procedure? And on the equipment used in processing? And on the records of operation and maintenance of that equipment? And, perhaps, on the computer systems that store and interpret those records?

Much like the layers in an onion, regulatory attention focuses over time at the earlier, inner steps of preparation and process, always moving backward to more proximal causalities of safety threats and problems. In part, that movement is a function of satisfaction with the more surface levels of control; in part it is a function of deeper understanding of the ultimate causes of problems. Arguably, an underlying causality of the trend derives from the reality that once investigators have achieved a satisfactory level of control for a surface issue, they have the time and resources to delve deeper; few regulators are likely to announce that the problem originally defined is now solved and that their agency or position is no longer necessary. But most significantly the trend to move backward to proximal causality is a response to consumer demand: Standards of cleanliness are continually raised in response to public understanding. The same trend applies to the performance (and absence of side effects) of drugs, the reliability and therapeutic value of medical devices, the purity of biologics, and the quality and safety of all other FDA-regulated products and processes.

At some point, of course, the costs associated with growing demands reach a point at which cost becomes a limiting factor. Human blood provides an illustrative example. While most transfusion blood donors are unpaid, there is a cost associated with collection. As screening costs rise, the resulting expense involved in providing a qualifying pool of product rises proportionately. In a simplistic example, if it costs $1 to collect a bag of blood, and only one in ten bags pass the screening criteria, the base cost per useable bag is $10. If those screening steps significantly increase the public health and safety, they are well worth any reasonable cost. But if the screening begins to provide only minimal value, shall we exclude anyone who has visited the United Kingdom in the last six months? In the last year? Who has shared a meal with anyone who visited the United Kingdom? The incremental cost of each bag can begin to act as its own rationing factor, deriving the poor (or the poor selectors of insurance) from desirable treatment.

To avoid such a situation requires that, at some point, a risk assessment is used to weigh the value of further testing or screening against the relative safety gain (and increased cost) of that process. Regulators have always dealt with these equations: How many adverse reactions are acceptable for a drug that provides valued therapy? Should a vaccine that can save thousands in the (possible) event of a disease outbreak, but that causes severe life-threatening complications in a small number of cases, be widely administered? How does that equation change if the disease event is increasingly likely? If the complications are increasing severe, or increasingly common?

The **risk assessment**, the balancing of increased safety against the limited effect of the cost of implementing that safety factor, is the second major regulatory trend. Originating in the review of medical devices, the concept of risk (or hazard) analysis considers the probability and potential severity of an adverse patient reaction, system performance, or manufacturing process. Regulatory scrutiny is then assigned, and supporting evidence collected, in proportion to the degree of risk inherent in a given situation.

The risk assessment represents a rational triage of regulatory energies, along with an assignment of the expense involved in a major regulatory study to those areas of highest concern. The effect is general lowering of noncritical regulation, combined with a slight, albeit real, reduction in ultimate drug prices. As drug prices are increasingly criticized, and as the FDA's budget is stretched even thinner, this rational approach to apportioning regulatory efforts represents a significant trend.

The third major trend may surprise many members of the general public and even some long-term industry practiners: The FDA has long and consistently declared that it does not regulate in pharma industries. Rather, the FDA has taken the consistent position that the industry is **self-regulated** and that the agency's job is to oversee and police this self-regulation.

All companies and products falling under the wide FDA umbrella are subject to internal quality assurance requirements. Even if a product performed flawlessly, without any side effects, purity defects, or adverse reactions, the manufacturer would be justly criticized if it did not have an appropriate quality assurance program in place. Anticipating the TQM and ISO 9000 movements of the 1990s, the FDA and its industries have long established a goal of not just the equivalent of zero defects, but of a quality system to continually improve and oversee the minimization of problems.

Working in conjunction with the proximity causality and risk assessment trends, this emphasis on self-regulation results in a continuing shift of attention backwards in the laboratory and manufacturing processes. Users of Laboratory Information Management Systems (LIMS) now routinely investigate their software suppliers, since the internal quality of an automated laboratory is dependent increasingly on the accuracy of the software that manages and interprets experimental results. In much the same way, manufacturers extend their quality assurance reach to vendors of raw materials, of manufacturing equipment, and of software control systems. The self-regulation, tempered by a risk assessment to put priority on areas of greatest potential danger, forces a proximal causality shift.

9.3   A DRUG EXAMPLE

The FDA regulatory process applies to all aspects of the process of bringing drugs from laboratory to consumer—except, sometimes, the discovery and development process. The drug discovery and development process is much like a sieve, testing many compounds to select the few promising solutions that will enter the formal testing to production pipeline. The majority of those compounds, never patented and never pursued, are in practice except from all regulation. Only those substances which continue on to an FDA Investigatory New drug (IND) filing and, hopefully, to preclinical and clinical testing and eventual manufacture and distribution are included in the regulatory process.

However, if a drug does continue on through the pipe line, there is a retrospective inclusion of its discovery and development under the regulatory umbrella. In reality, then, only successful drugs are subject to regulation in the discovery stage, but developers are forced to prepare all prospective drugs for that eventual regulation. This "retrospective regulation" is another example of the self-regulated nature of the industry. A research organization anticipating producing a successful drug is wise to implement its own regulatory program from inception in order to prepare for the eventual review of regulatory documentation for the few surviving compounds.

The self-regulation of drug discovery, in anticipation of possible regulatory review should a drug be the subject of an eventual IND, is further complicated by a recently evolving development. A number of drugs are tested for a specific purpose, and they fail to meet the standards for further investment. Later, that rejected drug is found to have a secondary effect for which it does represent a viable product. For example, Viagra may have proven not be the optimal solution to a search for a blood pressure reduction agent, but when reconsidered for a secondary "quality of life" condition emerged as a very successful product.

The reconsideration of rejected compounds again suggests self-regulation of the discovery process, to assure supporting documentation for all compounds regardless of their immediate promise. In almost all situations the most successful and cost-effective strategy is to operate the drug discovery and development process in accordance with regulatory guidelines, anticipating the possibility of eventual retrospective regulation.

There is significant exception. In the past, research universities have concentrated on basic research. In recent years, however, with the rise of technology transfer units in the major universities and the acceptance of entrepreneurship among science faculty, it has become not unusual for an academic research team to pursue the process through product development and licensure (and, in a few cases, formation of a company to bring the drug to market). The effect of incorporating the drug discovery and development process into the university setting is two fold.

First, traditionally and practically, university laboratories have been exempt from regulation. While this separation may have to be re-thought in the future, there are no immediate plans for FDA review of academic research facilities; and there are few, if any, plans by universities to conform to the record keeping, training, and testing requirements of the FDA. In effect the regulatory process for drugs developed in academic settings stops at the patent/licensure point.

Second, this separation places greater pressure on licensees—the drug companies—to themselves review not only the results of drug development, but also the controls and laboratory conditions that produced those results. University technology transfer offices are asked to produce Institutional Review Board records, as well as (increasingly) laboratory equipment records, certifications, and Installation Qualification/Operational Qualification records. While the FDA is unlikely to look at academic laboratories, the self-regulation of the industry is rapidly moving down to line. A university interested in maximizing the value of its licenses would be advised to include appropriate regulatory evidence in its portfolio documentation. Similarly, small start-up companies whose strategy relies on acquisition upon proof of product should include self-implemented regulatory review in their operations.

The effect of this self-regulatory trend in drug discovery and development is to suggest that while compliance may on the surface seem optional, the practical reality is quite different. If you are operating an unsuccessful discovery program, regulation is unnecessary. But if your plans include the hope that the program will ultimately lead to the development of successful products, then regulation, starting with self-regulation, is the only viable alternative.

Similarly, self-regulation is the assumption and key success strategy in medical device and biologics development. And the allocation of resources and priorities in that self-regulatory process is justified using a risk analysis.

9.4 BENEFITS ANALYSIS

A risk (or "hazard") analysis examines likely adverse scenarios and assesses the likelihood and severity of those scenarios. Missing from the assessment is a consideration of balancing "benefits" analysis. Consider, for example, a system that is designed to consolidate and interpret test blood processing test results. Presumably such a system would reject blood donation that exhibited evidence of HIV, hepatitis C, or other pathogens. But if a testing system reports trace levels of HIV—possibly a result of sample contamination, imprecise testing, or alternate sources of the enzyme used to indirectly measure the virus—should a blood donation be utilized? Prudence says no: If even a trace contaminant is measured, even if that trace is likely an anomaly, the donation should be rejected. The severity is simply too high to be an acceptable risk.

If the testing equipment is being validated, then, how should the regulatory risk be assessed? The probability of a misread—of declaring that no meaningful levels of HIV are identifiable when the sample actual contains a minute and insignificant trace—may be low, though the severity of such an error may be high.

But what if the blood donation—likely safe, but with a low chance of viral contaminant—is critically necessary? What if the alternative to the treatment is a higher probability of severity?

9.5 RISK ASSESSMENT

The risk assessment is the inverse coin of the benefits analysis. It examines the probability and severity of "negative" outcomes of a process, applicable to drug discovery, utilization of a pacemaker, manufacture of a drug, or any other process. In the regulatory world, however, a risk assessment has a unique role: it can help determine the amount of compliance evidence required for acceptance. In effect, a risk assessment of the drug discovery process (or any other process) can determine how closely the FDA will scrutinize, and how much time, energy, and expense should be dedicated to proving compliance.

To conduct a risk assessment, integrate these six steps into the process of planning and implementing a compliance strategy:

1. Utilizing the written requirement documentation for a specified system, device, computerized equipment, component or application, identify the desired performance under each of the defined requirement application.

2. Utilizing historical experiences with the specified system, device, computerized equipment, component, or application, and/or utilizing historical experiences related to predicate systems, devices, computerized equipment, components, or applications, and/or utilizing industry standards related to the specified system, device, computerized equipment, component or application, determine the alternate undesired performances for each defined requirement application.

3. For both the desired performance and the undesired performances for each defined requirement, determine the probability of occurrence each performance. Probability of occurrence can be calculated utilizing historical experiences with the specified system, device, computerized equipment, component, or application, and/or utilizing historical experiences related to predicate systems, devices, computerized equipment, components, or applications, and/or utilizing industry standards related to the specified system, device, computerized equipment, component, or application.

4. Analyze each of the undesired performances to characterize the severity of that performance in terms of risk to human life, health, and/or safety. "High severity" is generally defined as "loss of life, substantial loss of quality of life, and/or substantial disabling effect"; "medium severity" is generally defined as "compromise of quality of life, and/or some disabling effect"; and "low severity" is generally defined as "little or no effect on quality of life or on normal life activities."

5. For each undesired result, calculate the risk according to the following grid:

Severity	Probability	Risk
High severity	High probablility	High risk
High severitly	Medium probablility	High risk
High severity	Low probability	Medium risk
Medium severity	High probability	Medium risk
Medium severity	Medium probabiity	Medium risk
Medium severity	Low probability	Low risk
Low severity	High probability	Medium risk
Low severity	Medium probability	Low risk
Low severity	Low risk	Low risk

6. Apply the table results to the Validation Protocol or policy to determine the appropriate level of testing and validation.

9.6   RISK ASSESSMENT AND REGULATION

In the process of regulating the biologics, medical device, or drug discovery process, the risk assessment provides a measure of degree of regulation. But to what does that regulatory scrutiny apply?

In the most basic sense, regulation is applied to all aspects of the development process. But two important caveats mitigate that reality. First, as described above, regulation of drug discovery is applied only retrospectively. That is, the end product and process are subject to FDA requirements only if the decision is made to move the discovered substance forward in the developmental process. Lines and paths that are abandoned or halted are not subject to regulatory review. Strategically, of course, that restriction may be of little practical value since all paths are considered potentially successful (or they would not have been initiated); most organizations therefore opt to integrate regulatory controls in anticipate of possible success.

The second caveat has a greater strategic and tactical value. While the FDA is interested in all aspects of drug discovery (with the degree and intensity as defined in the risk assessment), the practical focus for the past 10 years and the foreseeable future is upon the tools utilized in discovery. Regulatory attention focuses on the discovery tools to assess the process, just as an educator may try to judge a student's readiness to learn by assessing reading skills. The student's reading skills, as well as the drug discovery tools, are effective foci because they represent both fundamental elements in the process and historical indicators of potential problem.

Since the drug discovery process is largely based upon the use of complex systems—automated laboratory equipment, molecular modeling software, statistical analysis systems, and so on—those tools tend to be computers. And it is the very nature of computers that causes the most regulatory concern.

Computer systems are complex, based upon internalized and sometimes obscured decision rules. They are flexible, allowing multiple applications with appropriate changes in internal directions (programs). And, unlike more convention paper trails, computers can overwrite the changes made to those decision rules, directions, and even databases, often leaving little or no markers indicating that changes were made.

These characteristics, coupled with the industry's increased reliance on the use of computer systems, have led to a focusing of a significant portion of regulatory energy on the automated tools of the field. In the drug discovery arena where reliance on computers is particularly high, the major regulatory focus, mitigated by risk assessment, has been on the systems that collect, analyze, manipulate, and report. The result of that focus is the newest of the FDA regulations, 21 CFR Part 11, "Electronic Signatures and Electronic Archives."

Originally intended to define rules for accepting electronic signatures in lieu of human (paper) signatures on documents, Part 11 has been expanded to define virtually all aspects of computer control and of the regulation of computer systems. The requirement includes standards for documentation of the validation (testing and managerial control) of systems; of the training and operating procedure assistance to be provided to users; of security, change control, and disaster recovery assurances; and so on.

The Part 11 requirement provides guidance for control of the system tools used in the drug discovery process. In a very practical way, it serves as an outline of the FDA scrutiny of drug discovery. To the degree and depth defined by the risk assessment, FDA is concerned with the aspects of drug discovery defined in Part 11. Evidence of compliance represents an insurance policy providing confidence that, should a drug move along the pipeline to a New Drug Application (NDA), the Food and Drug Administration will accept supporting data from the first stages of the discovery process.

Here is a summary of the "state-of-the-art" regulatory expectation:

REGULATION CHECKLIST

To assure quality control and regulatory compliance a facility should document evidence of:

- A **Risk Assessment:** Determination of nondesired alternate outcomes and results of the drug discovery operation; calculation of the approximate probability of those occurrences, utilizing historical logs and/or results of predicate device operations; determination of the potential severity (in terms of direct threat to human health and safety) of those occurrences; and resulting categorization of the operation as low, medium, or high risk.

- If risk is determined to be low, other steps can be mitigated (limited testing in validation), eliminated (the vendor audit), or reduced (the PQ).

- A **Validation** of the operation, including:

  - **System validation** of all automated components, including documentation of system requirements and design; development of a trace matrix to assure proper testing to those requirements and design elements; development and exercise of appropriate test scripts; a review of the code itself; and an analysis of the Standard Operating Procedures in place to assure appropriate use, archive, disaster recovery, change control, and training.

- **Process validation**, focusing on possible contamination of media, equipment, and final product, including but not limited to bacterial contamination (both gram positive and gram negative), viral contamination, and material contamination.

- **Part 11 Audit:** If the system is automated, the FDA regulation 21 CFR Part 11 "Electronic Records and Electronic Signatures" is applicable. Part 11 emphasizes:
  - An audit trail to track all data changes
  - If electronic signatures are in use:
    - Dual confirmation of identity
    - Locking of document after signature
    - Unambiguous time/date stamp

- Archive (electronic and human readable) of all files
  - Control of data accuracy
  - Appropriate training

- Audit of **system vendor**, either by an independent "expert witness" certifying compliance with appropriate regulations or by the end-user organization. Key elements in the audit are the criteria utilized and the credibility of the auditor (hence the preference for independent experts who have detailed knowledge of the vendor system, and who have credibility for the regulatory agency).

- An **Installation Qualification (IQ)**, using preestablished standards to assure appropriate initial implementation of the system or systems. The IQ may be conducted by the vendor, by the end-user organization, or by a combination of both.

- Initial and periodic **Calibration**, in accordance with a metrology plan appropriate to the specific system or systems in use. Some systems are self-calibrating; a few others do not require recalibration after initial installation.

- **Operational Qualification (OQ)** and **Performance Qualification (PQ)**, sometimes performed separately and (in some circumstances and systems) combined. The OQ assures the system is ready for use; the PQ assures that it is appropriately in use.

- **Problem Report:** A system for reporting (and reviewing) any encountered malfunctions, necessary changes, or other problems.

STANDARD OPERATING PROCEDURE: VALIDATION RISK ANALYSIS

While a risk analysis has broad applications in applying a variety of FDA regulations, it is currently most commonly applied to validation issues. As 21 CFR Part

11 (above) illustrates, risk has been integrally included in the validation and control of computerized systems utilized in drug development, biologics, and medical devices. This SOP template for a Validation Risk Analysis demonstrates the application.

BACKGROUND

The validation of computer systems has been an FDA guideline since 1989 and is formalized as a requirement in 21 CFR Part 11. The first, and arguably most important, step in validating a system is the adoption of a Validation Standard Operating Procedure (SOP) that provides an outline and guideline for the study.

The SOP from Chapter 2 provides a model Standard Operating Procedure for System Validation, intended as a starting point. On the theory that it is easier to edit than create, this model SOP should be carefully reviewed, evaluated, and modified to suit the circumstances and situation of a biomedical organization.

SUMMARY

Risk assessment represents a valuable and significant cost-containment strategy, rapidly evolving to affect all aspects of FDA regulation. It represents an effective and defensible rationale for maximizing regulatory efforts where that effort makes a difference to public health and safety, an economizing in areas in which the import is insignificant.

The focus on the risk assessment process is based upon three general trends. First, there is a nature trend to move every backward in regulatory concern to causal levels, resulting in a focus on the computer system tools used in drug discovery. That focus is most strongly reflected in 21 CFR Part 11, which defines the evidence of compliance necessary to utilize systems and accept the analysis and data that those systems provide.

Second, the intensity of the focus on systems (and on all other regulatory aspects) is tempered by a rational understanding that the significance of a danger should help define the degree of control of that danger. Cost controls suggest that investing in the collection of evidence or in expensive retesting should be mitigated by an analysis of the danger that an error represents. The result is the risk assessment, a tool used to determine the depth of control and of compliance evidence necessary. If Part 11 tells a drug discovery lab what will be examined in an FDA visit, the risk assessment predicts (a) the likelihood of that visit and (b) the depth or duration of the scrutiny involved.

The final trend lies in the origins of the FDA and its self-defined (and appropriate) role. The agency doesn't directly regulate. Rather, the FDA defines its role as supervising the self-regulation of an industry whose economic and altruistic interests require high levels of quality control. The drug discovery process should be and is self-regulated: The FDA's role is to assure the quality and consistency of that self regulation.

So Part 11 directs the focus to the system tools that control the process of drug development and discovery. The risk assessment determines the intensity of that beam. And an understanding of the self-regulated nature of the industry defines the real regulators.

The risk assessment process is appropriately regulated by drug discovery organizations, providing controls and evidence to a depth defined by a risk assessment, in accordance with standards defined in Part 11.

The following study suggests a model for apply risk analysis to the probability of an FDA site visit. It has been accepted by representatives of several FDA regions, with strong hints that the model is now used to select visitations sites, making it a deterministic as well as predictive tool.

A HEURISTIC MODEL OF FDA RISK FACTORS FOR CGMP INSPECTIONS OF PHARMACEUTICAL MANUFACTURING SITES[1]

Abstract

The United States Food and Drug Administration utilizes a diagrammatic model to explain subjective decisions for prioritizing cGMP inspections of pharmaceutical manufacturing sites. This heuristic model converts that series of diagrams and criteria into a mathematical formula that can be used to make key decisions about the design and quality control of a site to minimize the probability, duration, depth, and frequency of FDA visits (copyright Tikvah Therapeutics, Inc. of Atlanta, Georgia, USA, 2006). All rights reserved. Permission granted for duplication and distribution with attribution.

Background

Resource limitations affecting the US Food and Drug Administration have forced the agency to ration the domestic drug manufacturing venue inspections mandated to occur every two years. In the response the Agency's cGMPs for the 21st-Century Initiative pilots the use of a risk-based prioritization system for non-cause (routine) inspections. This pilot model identifies general variables and their relative significance, but stops short of providing a utilitarian heuristic model that mathematically expresses the relationships and weights of those variables. A heuristic mathematical model provides three potential advantages. First, such a model could be utilized to unambiguously rank and schedule future FDA visits. The result would be a tool for the measurement of efficiency and policy compliance of the agency in meeting its redefined burden of conducting at least high-risk inspections on a regular schedule. Second, the model could provide the pharmaceutical industry with some advanced warning of a pending inspection. Since inspections are intended to be snapshots of best practices, such a warning system would allow internal Quality Assurance

[1]Dr. Sandy Weinberg and Carl A. Rockburne.

departments to maximize the effective use of their resources and to plan (at least on a gross scale) for forthcoming regulatory events. Third, and of greatest interest to newly emerging pharma companies and to established companies in the process of designing and launching new facilities and operations, the model could improve effective planning, permitting energy and resources to be most efficiently allocated to quality issues. Knowing the FDA risk formulae would not only assist in the mundane task of anticipating FDA visits, but would also assist in the more important function of design of facilities and systems to minimize those factors that experience has shown are the most risky in terms of quality (rather than simply in terms of FDA attention). It is with this last value in mind that this paper attempts to construct a heuristic model of risk ranking for cGMP inspections of pharmaceutical manufacturing sites.

Variables

Fourteen (14) variables have been identified from FDA literature and are defined below:

Severity (S): The short-term effect of an undesired outcome, characterized as "death," "prolonged hospitalization," "acute illness," or "quality of life."

For each likely but undesired outcome, determine the most serious potential effect on human patients. Score: 4 = death; 3 = prolonged hospitalization; 2 = acute illness; 1 = compromised quality of life; 0 = none of the above.

Probability of Occurrence (P): The likelihood of a specific undesired outcome occurring based upon experience across companies and products.

For each likely but undesired outcome, determine based upon cross-industry experience the likely probability of occurrence. Score: 3 = high, occurs at or greater than once per five (5) production batches (20%); 2 = medium, occurs in fewer than once per five (5) production batches but at or rarer than once per twenty (20) production batches; 1+ less frequent than once per twenty (20) production batches.

History of Violation (V): Previous FDA findings of problems or nonconformities.

For the facility, Score: 3 = FDA has identified significant violations on a previous visit, resulting in sanctions; 2 = FDA has identified significant violations not resulting in sanctions; 1 = FDA has identified minor violations; 0 = FDA visit did not result in any findings of violations.

History of Inspection (I): Duration between FDA visits.

For the facility, Score: 3 = FDA has visited within last three years and has identified significant violations; 2 = FDA has not visited within the last three years; 1 = FDA has visited within the last three years and found no significant violations.

Volume of Material (VM): Amount of production material generated by a facility or facility subsystem.

For the facility, Score: 3 = production volume exceeds norm average; 2 = production facility approximates norm average; 1 = production volume below norm average (pilot facility).

Type of Establishment (T):   Product developer; manufacturer; contract manufacturer, repacker, etc.
Score: 3 = facility of contract manufacturer; 2 = facility is repacker; 1 = facility is manufacturing operation of licensed product developer.

Formulation (F):   Experience of problems or complications in the formulation of the product, including but not limited to separation issues, interactions, and/or subformulations.
Score: 3 = Significant formulation problems or complications experience, with most issues resolved; 2 = significant formulations problems encountered, with all issues resolved; 1 = no significant formulation problems encountered.

Sterility (St):   Complications in the process of assuring that product has no contaminants, such as filtration, heating, or filling issues.
Score: 3 = Significant sterility problems or complications experience, with most issues resolved; 2 = significant sterility problems encountered, with all issues resolved; 1 = no significant sterility problems encountered.

Cleanliness (C):   General environmental conditions that might lead to contamination or reduce the likelihood of same.
For the facility, Score: 3 = significant unchecked cleanliness issues; 2 = minor unchecked cleanliness issues; 1 = no unchecked cleanliness issues.

Dosage (D):   Complications related to the safe and proper dosage of the product, such as a narrow range of effectiveness, close-to-range negative reactions, and so on.
Score: 3 = Significant dosage problems or complications experience, with most issues resolved; 2 = significant dosage problems encountered, with all issues resolved; 1 = no significant dosage problems encountered.

Manufacturing Processes (M):   Complications related to complex manufacturing process, such as mixing, separations, and so on.
Score: 3 = Significant manufacturing processes problems or complications experience, with most issues resolved; 2 = significant manufacturing processes problems encountered, with all issues resolved; 1 = no significant manufacturing processes problems encountered.

Delivery Oversight (O):   Over the counter versus prescription versus hospital administered.
Score: 3 = over-the counter, without direct or indirect professional oversight; 2 = prescription required, providing indirect professional oversight; 1 = directly administered and overseen by professionals.

Environmental Issues (E):   Heat, pollution, air particulates, or other environmental factors likely contributing to product contamination.

For the facility, Score: 3 = significant environment issues existing; 2 = minor environmental issues; 1 = no environmental issues.

Quality Controls (Q):   The presence of quarantine, product checks, or other quality control functions.

Score: 4 = no significant quality controls in place; 4 = only end of process quality controls in place; 2 = only continuous process quality controls in place; 1 = continuous process and end of process quality controls in place.

Weighted Model

The 14 described above have been weighted based upon analysis of experiences with 138 FDA inspection case studies over the period 1999–2005. The model provides both (a) guidance concerning the likelihood of an FDA inspection and (b) the appropriateness of an FDA inspection. That is, it answers the question of whether or not the FDA is likely to visit, and of whether or not the FDA should schedule a visit. Furthermore, the model provides recommendations concerning the self-regulatory steps appropriate to minimizing the need for FDA intervention. As a heuristic tool, the model should be continuously modified and the relative weights of variables tweaked to reflect growing experience.

$$Y = ((5*\mu S) + (5*\mu P) + (3*V) + (2*I) + (Vm) + (T) + (2*F) + (2*St) + (C)$$
$$+ (2*D) + (M) + (2*O) + (E))*(Q) \qquad \text{High Score: 356} \qquad \text{Low Score: 20}$$

Range: Priority of FDA inspections

  0–125 Low   126–250 Medium   251–356 High

Caveat

This model includes only the 14 variables described by the FDA in their own literature. Other factors—change in management, company acquisition, new facility design, corporate culture, an so on—probably have significant impacts upon the probability of FDA inspections, but are not included here because the FDA has never formalized their influence on scheduling decisions. No doubt future improvements of the model should include these and other unofficial factors.

Applications

The model has four distinct applications, each appropriate to a different stakeholder. For FDA District Offices, the model can be used to prioritize and select sites for investigational visits. With appropriate adjustments over time, it will identify those facilities that maximize relative risk factors potentially compromising public health and safety. The model not only can serve to supplement or direct decision making processes regarding investigational priorities, it but also can rationalize those processes providing defensible criteria and consistent policy over time and across districts. With continuing tweaking and heuristic improvement, the model can assist the FDA in the management of stagnant and shrinking inspection budgets and in coping with always limited regulatory resources even as public demands and potential sites expand.

For established companies, the model can provide a template for continuous self-regulation and improvement. It clearly demonstrates the value of a rigorous quality assurance operation and of effective risk management of products and processes. With heuristic modification over time, the model can assist established companies in the allocation of internal resources and in the anticipation and management of external regulatory involvements. For emerging companies, the model can assist in the evaluation and selection of products and product applications, as well as in the design of quality assurance controls. To the extent that increased external regulatory involvement translates into increased costs and business risks, it can assist in comparing multiple production approaches and product selections. Again, the model is heuristic and must be tweaked based upon experience over time, but with that tweaking it can be added to business forecasting models and market projects to aid in rational decision-making.

For consulting and auditing operations, the model provides a tool for anticipating and quantifying potential client concerns. If included in a gap analysis, the model can quantify regulatory risks and be utilized to recommend control strategies to minimize those risks. The broach base of varying clients will provide heuristic data for further improvement of weighting and variable definition criteria, continually honing the model and increasing its value (in effect providing a clear added value over competing consulting organizations).

All of these applicational advantages flow from the heuristic nature of the model and its ability to grow and improve with experience.

Summary

The FDA Risk Factors Model is designed to provide a rational approach to anticipation and planning for cGMP inspections of pharmaceutical manufacturing sites. The model is heuristic in design, based initially on analysis of 138 recent inspections. With further experience over time, the relative weighs of the variables will be refined, and both the predictive and analytical value of the model will improve. Using this early version, it is possible to efficiently and rationally classify a particular manufacturing site as "high," "medium," or "low" risk. These categories can provide FDA officers with guidance in scheduling investigations; can provide established companies with recommendations for maximizing internal controls to smooth those visits; can provide emerging companies with guidelines for the selection of products, processes, and control elements; and can provide internal and external consulting operations with a tool for anticipating and coping with FDA investigations. The model utilizes the 14 variables currently described in the FDA literature. Over time, some variables are likely to prove redundant; some weight is likely to shift and is likely to reduce and simplify even as it improves in predictive value.[2] Or, in a continuous production operation, substituting "24 hours of production run" for "batch" experience with similar heuristic models suggests that over time and experience some variables will become redundant as analytical and predictive tools, and can be eliminated. Mature models are generally much more rigorous and much less complex than this early attempt which utilizes all fourteen variables identified in FDA literature.

The next article presents a heuristic model to explain the four-part process of the successful regulatory submission application.

REGULATORY RISK FINDINGS: PREDICTING FDA ACTIONS ON DRUG REGULATORY SUBMISSIONS[3]

Abstract

The outcomes of drug regulatory submissions to the US Food and Drug Administration often seem to be unpredictable. Some applications sail through without question; others are delayed; still other are rejected for reasons that may seem obscure or insignificant. As with any planned endeavor, and especially in the high technology realm of drug development, unexpected actions are a bane to effective planning, securing finance, and managing development. Using an evolving heuristic formula, the questions naturally arising in this environment may be answered. Can we predict the outcome? Can we maximize a positive result? Can we open the "black box?"

Introduction

The process of new drug development is highly structured with the US Food and Drug Administration following its mandate to protect the public and oversee the development and introduction of new pharmaceutical products. From the Investigational New Drug stage to New Drug Application, the submissions by pharmaceutical companies are often characterized by frustrating unpredictability.

Utilizing an evolving heuristic model, it is possible to gather more confidence in success based on expectations of positive FDA actions to these regulatory submissions.

---

[2]"Pharmaceutical CGMPs for the 21st Century: A Risk Based Approach," USFDA, 21 August 2002. "Risk-Based Method for prioritizing CGMP Inspections of Pharmaceutical Manufacturing Sites—A Pilot Risk Ranking Model," USFDA, September 2004. "Risk-Based Method for prioritizing CGMP Inspections of Pharmaceutical Manufacturing Sites—A Pilot Risk Ranking Model," US FDA, September 2004, and Revised API Inspection Compliance Program Guidance Manual CP 7356.002F, and Knisky, D. M., "Comparative Risk Projects: A Methodology for Cross-Project Analysis of Human Health Risk Rankings," August 1999.

[3]Dr. Sandy Weinberg, Clayton State University; and Dr. Ron Fuqua, Clayton State University.

The Reviews

The overall process involves four reviews: logistics, basics, controversy, and consensus. During the review of logistics, the FDA administrative staff is most important. Their responsibility is to check conformity to all requirements for the submission. If the application does not conform in all aspects, minor and major, the result can be rejection or delay, including the return of the application for resubmission.

Once the logistics of the submission have been confirmed, the application is assigned for basic review. The basic review can be described with these steps:

- Review by staff member (generally junior)
- Possible clarification questions
- Reference to Pre-Submission Meeting memo
- Delays if amendments are required
- Pass to senior reviewer if controversial issues are identified
- Pass to committee when complete

The review for controversy issues result in a request for more information. It is better to identify the controversy prior to submission, ideally in discussion at the Pre-Submission Meeting, and to resolve the issue in advance of review.

The consensus review is conducted by the FDA review committee. The preliminary and secondary reports are reviewed. The application document itself is scrutinized. The opportunity to question exists and affords the final opportunity to resolve any outstanding issues.

This four-part review—logistic, basic, controversy (if necessary), and consensus committee—creates a virtual black box process. With a clear understanding of the stages and procedures, end decisions may seem arbitrary and unpredictable.

In reality, however, it is possible to construct a preliminary heuristic model that can provide a clear insight into likely end decisions.

The Model

The model consists of 10 variables that are developed and evaluated during the four reviews. A three-point scale (high, medium, low) avoids the requirement for fine distinctions and allows a simple, straightforward assignment of value to each variable. While the model is heuristic and still evolving as additional data are gathered and analyzed, the weights for each variable are proving functionally predictable of success for the FDA submission when a resulting score is 30 or higher.

During the four steps of review already described, 10 variables are produced. These are:

- S = success defined
- R = pre-review
- D = follow directions (conformity to all logistical requirements)
- P = Follow pathways (utilization of standardized and widely acceptable study designs)

- B = reButtals (development of reasoned and supported responses to controversial issues)
- H = history (experience with related molecules and drugs)
- T = poliTics (media and public demands for rapid approval, increased safety, etc.)
- J = preJudices (personal preferences and concerns of major FDA committee members)
- V = diVision (Neurology, Metabolic, and other FDA Divisions, and their foci)
- L = leadership (experience and expertise of the FDA committee chair and division head)

The current heuristic formula, applied to the variables after they are scored on a three-point scale, is

$$\text{Approval score} = f\{(2{*}S) + (5{*}R) + (3{*}D) + (2{*}P) + (3{*}B)$$
$$+ (H) + (2{*}T) + (J) + (2{*}V) + (2{*}L)\}$$

By predefining success, you are able to develop a clear definition of a likely outcome. If necessary, additional studies can be done and cost factors identified. Using pre-reviews allows an FDA simulation and an opportunity to identify early any areas of controversy. It also allows the opportunity to prepare summary reports that can be used as rebuttal. To follow directions implies the elimination of doubts before submissions by asking questions, reading FAQs, providing contact information, and avoiding deviations, even when considered insignificant.

Following pathways is similar to following beaten paths where those who have gone before have trod. In other words, avoid the mistakes of others and enjoy their successes. Model after accepted documents and avoid the desire to be creative, at least for the submissions. Use the most widely accepted methodologies and analyses. In preparing rebuttals, it is best if they can be kept informal. Avoid the appeals process when possible relying instead on informal requests for opportunities to provide additional information or to correct mistakes. Avoid using fairness, consistency, cost, or altruism arguments.

In the model, the last five variables are important as structural factors. The history variable is a hard lesson for some. Avoid the past mistakes of others by including history, considering politics, and knowing personal prejudices and preferences. Understanding where division exists in both opinion and style is useful to learn from history as well as recognizing the source of leadership in the agency with regard to your submission area.

Summary

The US Food and Drug Administration is responsible for new drug development review and approval. Its process is clearly delineated for those involved in the industry. Despite the clear outline of responsibilities and the well-known steps in the approval process, often submissions and their outcomes are not successful. Using this heuristic model, the results of those submissions to the FDA may become more predictable. With that predictability comes (a) the ability to fine-tune the submission application and (b) an increased probability of success. The benefits of establishing a strong internal pre-review process, using the model as an evolving guideline, can enhance successful outcomes from an otherwise confounding black box.

CHAPTER 10

CASES

The cases described in this chapter provide examples of the ways in which the six strategies for regulatory cost containment have been effectively applied in the pharmaceutical, medical device, and biologics industries.

These cases are real, taken from the files of over 25 years of consulting to and advising executives in the industry. Obviously, details have been changed, obscured, or eliminated to protect confidential relationships.

Special thanks are due to three fellow consultants who contributed particularly illustrating cases:

Dr. Ronald Fuqua of the Department of Health Care Management at Clayton State University

Mr. Arthur Spalding, Founding Partner of TAMM Net, Inc., a medical device consulting firm

Mr. Carl A. Rockburne, President of The Rockburne Group, regulatory consultants

Case Code: P1A

Case: Quality Systems Validation

Author: Weinberg

Industry: [X] Pharma   [ ] Biologics   [ ] Medical Device

Strategy: [ ] Requirements   [X] Audits   [ ] Quality by Design

[ ] Outsource   [ ] Electronic Submissions   [ ] EMEA Overlap

STRATEGIC ACTION

The organization has made the determination that (a) it cannot be dependent upon sporadic and often nonexpert FDA visits to assure that each of the 19 facilities appropriately follow system quality control procedures, (b) internal audits, while valuable, are not viewed with the same rigor as outside audits, and (c) the organization lacks the resources to assemble a highly credible, expert, experienced audit team that can visit all 19 sites on a regular (semiannual) basis.

Cost-Contained Regulatory Compliance: For the Pharmaceutical, Biologics, and Medical Device Industries, First Edition. Sandy Weinberg.
© 2011 John Wiley & Sons, Inc. Published 2011 by John Wiley & Sons, Inc.

Therefore:

(a) The company hires an outside audit team with a strong track record of FDA acceptance of its Expert Opinion, with specific expertise with computer systems used in quality assurance and control, with large molecule production systems, with international pharmaceutical regulation, and with a history of more than 20 previous comparable audits. The team is charged with the development of a set of audit standards, the training of local staff and dissemination of those standards, and the semiannual audit of each facility to assure compliance with the established standards.

(b) The company convenes a multi-day meeting of representatives of each of the facilities, including computer systems personnel, qa/qc personnel, and manufacturing personnel, chaired by the outside audit team, to develop specific audit standards.

(c) The company schedules on-site two-day training programs at each of the facilities (actually, at 11 facilities, combining staffs of co-located facilities) to familiarize all relevant staff with the new audit standards. Training is conducted in English (the company language) with translated lecture slides and notes available in Spanish, French, German, and Chinese.

(d) Three months after the last training course, the company begins an ongoing process of auditing each site with an unannounced visit of approximately 3 days' duration, assuring semi-annual audits of all facilities. A master report, including the standards, training program, project SOP, and all of the 19 audit reports, is retained at the company headquarters and is reviewed by the corporate VP for Quality on an annual basis. A site report, including the standards, training program, project SOP, and all site Audit Reports, is retained at each site and is reviewed by the facility Director of QA/QC on an annual basis.

The direct costs of this audit program (standards development; 11 training programs; 10 annual audits) were a total of $225,000. Indirect costs, including travel expenses, employee training time, and so forth, was estimated at an additional $250,000 in year one (training courses) and $150,000 per year in subsequent years. A 3-year complete cycle (standards development, training, audit of all 19 sites) therefore totals $1,225,000.

Savings against this total include avoidance of FDA criticism, possible recall, subsequent damage control, and a negotiated reduction in corporate liability (self-) coverage of $2 million per year, resulting in a direct savings of $5,775,000.

EFFECT

The effect of the development of a comprehensive audit program for the global computerized quality assurance and control system was a leadership role in the industry and in the regulatory community. The approach, the audit standards, and the training/review process became the model to which the FDA pointed when critiquing other systems and controls. And, with semiannual audit certificates and reports issued by an outside credible and expert auditor group, the FDA never criticized (or, for that matter, conducted more than a cursory review of) the computerized system. More importantly, the second (audit) look at the operation of the system in accordance with a set of clear audit standards (and hence second checking the internal preparation for the randomly occurring audits) prevented, over the 12 years of the program, any serious problems that could have resulted in product recall or in release of unsafe product.

At the end of the 10-year relationship the organization replaced the global qa/qc system and determined that it had developed sufficient in-house expertise and credibility to replicate the audit program without the need for outside personnel. The process of jointly developing standards was repeated, site personnel were trained, and a semi-independent audit team began a visitation schedule at all (now 17) sites. Every three years the leader of the original outside audit team is invited in for a review and critique of the process to assure conformity with the project SOP.

The effect of this outside audit strategy has been the highest level of quality control and assurance; FDA acknowledgement of that high level; and the eventual development of that credibility in house.

PROBLEMS/CHALLENGES

The two major problems encountered in the project can both be characterized as "drift." The first, a personnel issue, applies to the audit team: while the audit leader was able to assure stable review over the 10 years of operation, there was significant turn over in the other team members (a total of six persons acted as audited assistants over the timeframe), largely as a result of their enhanced value of this system was replicated in other organizations and they became leaders of teams of their own. Second, with 19 sites using the same software, there is a drift in the systems that results from minor changes, fixes, and enhancements over the years. By year 10, the system not only has evolved from its original code, but some of the 19 sites had evolved in different subtle by significant directions. This process made the audits more cumbersome, and the use of audit standards more important. In a post-project critique, however, it was suggested that future projects should have a 5-year rather than 10-year lifespan to minimize the system drift (and, perhaps, to reduce the human team drift as well).

COST CONTAINMENT

The direct project cost containment largely came from increased corporate confidence in the accuracy and credibility of quality data reported by the 19 systems, permitting a reduction in the liability underwriting and reserves. While for the initial 10 years there was some cost containment realized by the use of part-time expert auditors rather than full-time salaried and benefit-paid employees, the fact that the organization lacked the expert and credible personnel to conduct the audits itself makes this an impossible comparison and calculation.

Finally, there are unmeasured but real cost containment realized from the FDA enthusiastic acceptance of the scheme and from the avoidance of major recalls and problems. These savings may actually represent the largest portion of the gain despite their slippery nature. To some degree, however, the reduction in liability protection represents a recognition of this containment.

ESTIMATED SAVINGS

Direct: $5,775,000
Indirect: incalculable

NOTES

In addition to the liability reduction represented by a successful system audit, the organization gains signficiant indirect value. Without an audit, the review is conducted by the FDA on a sporatic visit: The result could be approval of full compliance, or a range of problems resulting in anything from a mild identification in a 483 through a signficiant finding with reaudit to a letter of warning to a product batch recall to a complete shutdown of the facility. With the audit conducted by an outside expert team, the same findings would result in a recommendation for correction, and ultimately (presumably) approval as compliant. The outside team avoids adverse actions, embarrassment, and potential fines.

While using an outside team provides credibility as well as expertise and experience, most organizations position themselves to eventually bring the audit function in house. Most commonly this is accomplished by adding one or more employees to the outside audit team, providing those persons with experience, training, and increased referred credibility.

Finally, the process of conducting an audit by a credible team of experts (outside or, eventually, in house) has a "spillover" effect on regulatory credibility. The FDA's preferred and appropriate role is a quality checker for a self-regulated organization; the audit is the ultimate demonstration of self-regulation.

Case Code: P1ES
Case: Electronic Filing Drug IND
Author: Weinberg
Industry: [X] Pharma   [ ] Biologics   [ ] Medical Device
Strategy: [ ] Requirements   [ ] Audits   [ ] Quality by Design
               [ ] Outsource   [X] Electronic Submissions   [ ] EMEA Overlap

BACKGROUND

The company is a start-up drug development organization focusing on neurological drugs, specifically aimed at the control of combat-related stress disorder (CRSD), a variant of post-traumatic stress disorder. A promising molecule has been licensed from a nearby research university: Preliminary preclinical research has been conducted, and key published studies have been investigated. The next major step is the preparation of an Investigatory New Drug (IND) application.

A traditional IND runs about 30 notebook volumes (mostly containing copies and reviews of published studies) and costs about $300,000 of in-house time (or outside consulting fees). After discussions and a pre-submission meeting with the appropriate FDA review team, the company has determined that there are three submissions options:

Option One. The "traditional" all paper submission.

Option Two. A modified paper submission: traditional paper, plus an electronic copy with hyperlinks to an indexing system.

Option Three. A fully electronic submission.

Without being explicit, the FDA seems to be encouraging option two (the modified paper with hyperlink copy). It is, however, the most expensive option, estimated at about $450,000 (in effect, both a paper and an electronic preparation). The fully electronic copy (Option Three) is estimated at $250,000—about the same preparation time, but less labor in photocopying and assembling multiple copies of the 30 notebooks.

Under standard FDA guidelines the agency has 6 months from filing to review an IND and raise any suggestions or objections before the submitter is permitted to proceed with the proposed study(s). Electronic, hybrid, and paper copies must all be reviewed within the same 6-month timeframe.

STRATEGIC ACTION

The organization determined that the post-cost-effective submission scheme was the electronic submission (Option Three). The electronic submission would save further time and expense in the future when the New Drug Application (NDA) was filed. And the FDA was at least nominally comfortable with the concept of an electronic review based upon the suggestions from the agency concerning the hybrid (Option Two) submission. Wishing to maintain a positive working relationship with the FDA, however, and realizing that some of the agency review team members seem uncomfortable with an entirely electronic submission (despite FDA guidelines), the company communicates two offers to the FDA: to provide one day of training/assistance to the FDA team members what might be unfamiliar with or uncomfortable with the relatively new electronic submission format and/or to provide a single unofficial paper copy of the IND core (the application with supporting bibliography but without paper copies of all of the reviewed publications: approximately two notebooks in total). After due consideration, the agency rejected (with thanks) both offers and decided to rely entirely on the electronic submission.

The IND was reviewed within the 6-month framework and was approved without significant question, condition, or revision.

By adopting the electronic submission strategy with organization, we realized an immediate savings of $50,000 over the paper alternative (Option One), or $200,000 over the hybrid (Option Two). More significantly, by organizing the IND in electronic format, the organization prepared for three important future cost savings:

1. The electronic IND paved the way for FDA acceptance of an electronic NDA at the successful conclusion of the clinical testing and analysis. That NDA document is much more time-sensitive (FDA delays result in significant loss of patent protection and hence drug valuation).

2. The preparation of the future electronic NDA is eased and to some degree expedited by the availability of the IND content in electronic form, resulting in greater savings from the three options of NDA submission.

3. The availability of the IND (and, ultimately, the NDA) in electronic form allows simple reformatting and modification for simultaneous submission to EMEA (see Chapter 6), a further significant cost-containment strategy.

The direct savings ($50,000 to $200,000) were dwarfed in this case by indirect savings in the form of more rapid assembly and approval of the NDA (having the effect of expanding the effective patent life) and permitting the rapid modification of the IND (and, eventually, the NDA) to the EMEA format, permitting simultaneous submission to both agencies. While indirect savings are not currently calculable (the NDA is still some years away), the potential indirect cost containment is likely to be sizeable.

EFFECT

In an established company where procedures, staffing, and resources for the management and production of massive paper documents may be well in place, the generation of a paper IND may represent routine. In fact, the production of an electronic submission may represent a radical departure of procedure, requiring some extra investment of energy, time, and resources. Since a new organization is in effect inventing itself, adoption of the Option Three all electronic submission is an appropriate choice: There is no question that the FDA is phasing in electronic submissions, and it is reasonable to predict that manual submissions will be obsolete (and, perhaps, unacceptable) within the next 5–10 years. Electronic systems are increasingly reliable; FDA and industry staffs are increasingly familiar with the use and advantages of an electronic submission, and the electronic tools for cross-reference, hyperlinking, searching, and other functions are growing in convenience and accessibility. In the short run a company with a manual document control center may opt for paper submissions, but it would be difficult to justify the development of such an operation anew. Similarly, consulting organizations that rely heavily on the paper management capabilities for their competitive advantage will shortly find themselves with a shrinking market and an environment that little values their strength.

Well-designed, user-friendly, and effectively supported electronic submissions systems are less expensive to organize, easier to utilize, and more powerful in analytical capability. While formats are emerging and standards are in flux, there may be some reason to move slowly, but little doubt about how the future generally looks. Only a complete Luddite would expect that the advantages of electronic regulatory submissions will not outcompete paper alternatives in the evolutionary process.

PROBLEMS/CHALLENGES

In the past 3 years, electronic submission standards have gelled, and an increasingly clear picture of acceptable formats and features is emerging. That picture will continue to focus, but few if any revisions are to be expected.

The increasing use of electronic submissions has revealed a hidden weakness, however, that will probably be corrected in time to become a seventh cost-containment strategy in future editions of this book. Increasingly, the FDA is demanding (appropriately) that literature reviews be international in scope, and hence diverse in language. But the currently commercialized translation programs, particularly when faced with highly technical jargon, are generally inadequate. Presumably sometime in the future the FDA will require that non-English publications be accompanied by translations (an expensive process) or linked to effective translational software. That software is needed, as soon as possible.

COST CONTAINMENT

The direct cost containment was realized as a result of selecting the option of an electronic submission of the IND and reducing the paper workload and complexities of copying, assembling, and delivering the documents, as well as by avoiding the hybrid requirement of adding to that paper process an electronic (presumably scanned file) hyperlinked addendum.

Indirect cost containment will be realized in the future as the organization prepares and submits additional electronic documents using the same system, including a future (much more complex and extensive) NDA application. The electronic submission process not only conserves preparation resources but also saves time in both the preparation and review periods, translating into significant cost containment as elapsed time is deducted from patent protection—and hence marketing advantage.

ESTIMATED SAVINGS

Direct: $50,000–$200,000

Indirect: unable to calculate future indirect cost containment

NOTES

A significant percentage of the (paper) multiple pages of manual INDs consists of paper copies of published studies, photocopied and organized into notebooks. Because journals are increasingly published on line, however, the use of paper copies will represent yet another inefficient step in the assembly process. For electronic submissions, a hyperlink to the published article will take little effort. For paper copies, however, the electronic copy will be printed, copied, collated, assembled, and published. The relative cost savings gap will likely increase.

The side comment on translation software for published studies is exacerbated in the event of an EMEA submission. Some EMEA submissions—orphan drug applications, for example—are required to be submitted in all approved EMEA languages, a list that includes Icelandic, Finnish, and other languages uncommonly spoken in the United States. The challenge of translating an article originally published in Finnish into Icelandic for review by a native Italian speaker is mind boggling, but likely to be part of the process—much simplified by the inclusion with the submission of a link to effective translation software.

A Final Note: An acquaintance regulatory librarian was recently presented on retirement with a gold (plated) page numbering stamp, once the essential tool of the professional. One suspects that a new professional in the field would not recognize such a device even if encountered in a museum.

Case Code: B1E

Case: Laboratory Testing Software

Author: Weinberg

Industry: [X] Pharma   [ ] Biologics   [ ] Medical Device

Strategy: [ ] Requirements   [ ] Audits   [ ] Quality by Design

       [ ] Outsource   [ ] Electronic Submissions   [X] EMEA Overlap

BACKGROUND

This software development company, located in the Rocky Mountain region of the United States, is funded by and works in cooperation with a major international manufacturer of laboratory and manufacturing processing equipment. The systems are used by the Biologics industry, but the software itself is classified and regulated by FDA and EMEA as a medical device. The company has 26 employees (mostly programmers and software testing professionals), and has been ISO 9000 certified by KEMA Registered Quality.

Although the registration of software is not strictly enforced, the connection between this company and its funding parent has led to the decision to seek formal registration from both the FDA and EMEA. Furthermore, management has decided that FDA and EMEA approval will help differentiate the software in a crowded market and will provide potential customers with reassurance; some potential buyers have expressed skepticism about the small size of the company and the relatively small current user base.

The company's Vice President for Regulatory Affairs (Mary) runs a virtual department, relying on subcontractors and consultants to control documents, develop Standard Operating Procedures, and perform other regulatory functions: She coordinates those activities and acts as the final Quality Assurance reviewer for all regulatory and compliance responsibilities.

Mary has prepared two Requests for Proposal. The first RFP (#1A and #1B) asks consulting firms to bid on the development of an FDA 510(k) application; asks for approval to market a medical device in the United States, with contingent Pro-Market Approval data justifying no need for further clinical testing; and asks for a subsequent equivalent EMEA application, citing the (proved) FDA application as support.. The second RFP (#2) calls for the simultaneous development of both FDA and EMEA applications, tailoring the same data and arguments to both agencies but with different formatting and referencing/citation sections.

STRATEGIC ACTION

Mary's two RFPs have each been sent to three qualified consulting firms (total of six firms), selected on the basis of their previous histories of success with Medical Device applications to both FDA and EMEA; general reputation; resources; business history and credit report; and the backgrounds of the proposed staff members to be assigned to the project(s).

She has converted differing costing formulae (some firms bill hourly; others by the project; some add management fees, others build project management in; etc.) and averaged the proposals in both categories (sequential FDA and EMEA; simultaneous overlapping applications).

Before directly comparing financial proposals, Mary has noted four general strategic considerations:

- Sequential submissions allow the use of one approval to bolster and support the second application.
- Simultaneous application significantly reduces the review time (overlapping the FDA and EMEA review periods), speeding the time to market and reducing costs.
- Sequential applications ease the compliance management process, making Mary's job less complicated.
- Simultaneous application requires complex electronic formatting to manipulate application sections into appropriate order and location for each application.

These four factors will significantly affect Mary's final strategic decision.

The bids for two RFP produced the final adjusted averages:

Subsequent Submissions

FDA	$242,300.00
EMEA	$239,800.00
Subtotal	$482,100.00
Simultaneous Submission	$439,000.00

In this case, the simultaneous submission strategy resulted in a direct cost savings of approximately 10%.

Also important in Mary's decision, the simultaneous approach was likely (assuming successful approval) to reduce the review time by approximately 6 months, allowing a much more rapid global rollout of the product. Of course, Mary's final decision was balanced by the possibility under the sequential strategy that problems found by the FDA could be corrected in the EMEA application, increasing the probability of regulatory approval. If the FDA found problems under the simultaneous strategy, the likelihood of approval by both agencies was significantly reduced, and even approval by one agency was problematic.

EFFECT

The implementation of the simultaneous submission strategy is based upon the development of a database of application sections that can be rearranged and modified to meet the unique requirements of the FDA and EMEA. Once this database is defined and established, future simultaneous applications are significantly simplified.

The effect of the strategy is not only the relatively insignificant 10% savings between approaches (the range of bids on the RFPs within any one strategy exceeds the variance between the average bids of the two strategies: in direct savings, one would be better served with the not-so-profound advice of "select the lowest qualified bidder") but is also a more important time savings. The review period for an FDA or EMEA application is approximately six months each. Even with a longer one-time preparatory time (as opposed to separate preparations for the two agency applications), the adoption of a simultaneous strategy is likely to reduce the review by that nonoverlapping six months.

Calculating 120 working days for the additional six months of review, at an estimated average loss of revenue within patent period of $25 million USD per day, this strategy could produce a 20-year savings of $3 billion USD. While that figure may be highly optimistic in this case (the life span of software is more likely to be 2 years than 20), it is reasonable to estimate a potential market savings of approximately $150 million. Even this adjusted figure is optimistic: Given fluctuations in the software market, the relatively lower potential of medical devices versus pharmaceuticals, and some complications in the initial development of the simultaneous submission process, the company in case B1E estimates that their market savings using the simultaneous registration approach was approximately $12 million.

PROBLEMS/CHALLENGES

This organization faced three challenges. First, and most importantly, the EMEA and FDA definitions of predicate devices varied, forcing the company to accept the more conservative FDA definition for both applications (to simultaneously submit to both, it is necessary to default to the more conservative requirements). Second, initial establishment of sectional database required some time investment that should be recovered as new software versions are submitted: The first time learning curve was quick but did cause some delays. Finally, the company initially erred in the formatting of the two submissions, requiring a correction and resubmission of the FDA 510(k) and abbreviated PMA applications, losing approximately two weeks of review overlap. Estimated theoretical additional cost was approximately $1.5 million, resulting in a realized savings of approximately $10.5 million. All three of these problems were attributed to initial unfamiliarity with the simultaneous submissions approach and are expected to be eliminated in subsequent submissions. An after-action critique suggested using a consulting group familiar with the simultaneous submissions process to avoid these initial problems.

COST CONTAINMENT

Utilizing the simultaneous submissions strategy (FDA and EMEA), this organization was able to reduce the consulting costs of preparing medical device applications to the two regulatory agencies, but (much more importantly) was able to significantly reduce the total review time of the two applications, resulting in real potential savings through control of patent period and a competitive speed to market. Although not a historical part of this particular case, further cost containment could potentially have been realized through simultaneous submissions to regulatory agencies in Canada, Brazil, Israel, Australia, and Switzerland (Japanese formatting and regulations are sufficiently distinct as to make this approach highly problematic).

As with any new strategy, the organization found some difficulties with initial implementation that they expected (and subsequently have found) would be eliminated with greater experience with the approach.

ESTIMATED SAVINGS

Direct: $43,100
Indirect: $10.5 million

NOTES

Medical device software presents several cost-containment strategic challenges. First, all regulatory agencies are struggling with (a) their relative lack of experience and expertise and (b) the problem of software capababilities and applications evolving much more rapidly than regulatory standards. Second, savings resulting from the reduction of patent life due to regulatory delay are problematic given the relatively short lifespan of the product: It is unlikely that even the most sophisticated software will still be in use 8–10 years after introduction. The time savings therefore result more from the competitive advantage of speed to market than from increased longevity of patent protection. Third, the use of a new simultaneous submission strategy requires a learning curve on the part of consultants as well as companies: The combination of a consulting group bringing both experience in the strategy and expertise in the registration of software is a relative rarity.

As with all cost-containment strategies, the least effect will be seen with medical devices, simply because medical devices require the least capital to develop and represent the lower regulatory compliance allocation. Since the total expense is lower, the relative and proportionate cost savings realized is lower as well. Regardless, this company found significant savings in the simultaneous submission to both USFDA and EMEA of registration materials.

Case Code: B1O

Case: Supply Chain Analysis

Author: Weinberg

Industry: [X] Pharma   [ ] Biologics   [ ] Medical Device

Strategy: [ ] Requirements   [ ] Audits   [ ] Quality by Design

[X] Outsource   [ ] Electronic Submissions   [ ] EMEA Overlap

BACKGROUND

This case makes the direct calculation of cost containment a simple and accurate process. A global manufacturer of biologic monoclonals employed an in-house team to (among other responsibilities) conduct an annual analysis of the product supply chain to assure consistent temperature and pressure controls and to maintain sterility. Product sensitivity coupled with the vulnerability of patient made the annual analysis a critical compliance and control issue. Complications of the manufacturing and distribution process, involving steps in four countries and five different facilities, made the analysis particularly complex.

The team of three (led by SueAnne) spent approximately 30 persons days (90 days in total) following the product from initial production to patient use each year, testing and critiquing each intermediate step in the process. After 3 years of experience with this analysis, the company was purchased by a major conglomerate; and in the merger restructuring, SueAnne, the team leader, accepted a generous retirement package (the other two team members were assigned to other duties).

A few months later the VP for Manufacturing, Hans, contacted SueAnne and asked her to conduct the annual analyses as an outside consultant. SueAnne assembled a new team (recruiting two independent consultants to assist her) and continued to perform the same annual analysis.

By using a highly skilled and highly experienced team (or at least team leader) for a project of finite duration (about one month each year), the organization was able to effectively use outsourcing as a cost-containment strategy. The calculation of difference between the salary and benefits paid to SueAnne's in-house team and her outsource bid provides an accurate measure of the savings.

STRATEGIC ACTION

The organization made a major strategic shift post acquisition/merger in this and many other activities. In-house generalist employees were reassigned or reduced in number, and highly specialized employees requiring detailed expertise and experience were outsourced to established expert consultants. The annual Supply Chain Analysis function was an anomaly: The original plan was to move the function to outside experts, and the previous team leader was offered a generous retirement package (which she accepted with pleasure). When the time came to find an outside expert, however, it was determined that the same retired team leader—SueAnne— had developed the expertise and experience needed when she was an inside employee, and she was the most qualified external outsource consultant. Corporate policy prohibited utilizing an ex-employee as a consultant for a one-year period, but it was possible to schedule the next supply chain analysis just outside the one-year window, and SueAnne, assisted by her own outside consultants, accepted the contract.

SueAnne's team conducted a thorough analysis, following the product stream from facility to facility, testing for controls and purity and assuring adherence to company SOPs and regulatory guidelines and requirements. The outside team followed the same protocols that SueAnne had developed while serving as a full-time employee.

Note that SueAnne's consulting contract was fixed price (plus travel expenses), providing her with an incentive to be as efficient as possible while following the protocol. Her carefully selected outsource team—trained by SueAnne—moved rapidly, efficiently, and thoroughly.

When working in house, SueAnne and her team had been paid a total salary of $240,000, plus 32% overhead. The annual analysis project required 1.5 months for each of the team members:

In-house cost   ($316,000 annual: 1.5 months) $39,600

When working outside the corporation, freed from other responsibilities, meetings, and so on, SueAnne calculated that her team could perform the analysis in 20 days (60 person days). Therefore, SueAnne paid her two consultant team members $6000 each ($300 per day) and calculated her compensation at $750 per day ($15,000):

Outsource cost $27,000

Cost containment: savings $12,600, approximately 30%. Note that there were some additional savings in travel costs as the duration of the project is reduced. The savings realized are a direct effect of the "extra-organizational" status of the team, permitting a gain in project efficiency and in the reduction of overhead expenses. This highly specialized team, presumably selling its services to other biologics companies other months, leverages its expertise, experience, and regulatory reputation to efficiently perform analyses and assure cost-contained regulatory compliance.

EFFECT

Obviously the organization could potentially have retained SueAnne and would have realized the same benefit as she utilized her growing expertise and experience. As that expertise grew, however, the nonanalysis activities of her team the other 10.5 months of the year would have been increasingly inefficient use of their time. By using an outsource team—coincidentally led by the same person—the organization maximized the efficient use of SueAnne's talents. In addition, as she sold her specialized analysis skills to other companies the remaining months of the year, and in the process increased her experience, regulatory contacts, reputation, and expertise, SueAnne relative value as an outsource consultant increased. The effect, then, is a relatively small financial savings in absolute terms (a significant percentage) but a gain in quality of the annual supply chain investigations and the reliability of the assurance of compliance and control.

When taken in context as a general strategy for cost containment of regulatory compliance, the effect of assembling a series of ad hoc teams of highly specialized experts used as outsource resources and coordinated by a relatively small group of in-house generalists is a highly efficient and effective approach. While other cases will test the value of outsourced generalists retained on long-term contract, this small but powerful case demonstrates the effect of the adoption of an outsource cost-containment strategy that maximizes the use of specialized consultants.

The effect of the strategy on this multinational conglomerate corporation should be enhanced regulatory compliance, a highly (and increasingly) credible consultant conducting annual analyses, critical quality control of a highly vulnerable product, and cost containment.

PROBLEMS/CHALLENGES

There are three potential problems that should enter into the planning of the newly merged company. First, as SueAnne and her outside team increase their experience and regulatory credibility, their rates are likely to increase significantly. Since the value of their opinion will increase proportionately, the increase is probably justified, but the budget impact should be anticipated. Second, a specialized team or individual consultant is likely to be in high demand: Future availability may be a problem. And third, the shift from in-house to outsourced analysis of the supply chain in the likely to leave the company with an in-house lack of expertise applicable to other supply chain issues, such as redesign or new product development. Two recommendations can mitigate these problems. First, it may be advantageous to offer SueAnne a multi-year consulting contact, locking in a specific analysis month each year at a preset rate, controlling the likely cost increase and avoiding an availability issue. Second, the organization may consider having an in-house generalist accompany SueAnne's team through all or part of its analysis, preserving some level of in-house expertise and avoiding undue dependence.

COST CONTAINMENT

The shifting of a limited-duration highly specialized quality and regulatory function resulted in a reduction of the cost of that compliance activity of approximately 30%—a minor cash savings of approximately $12,600. The case does, however, permit a direct comparison of the benefits and costs of an in-house versus an outsource team conducting identical tasks.

Arguably under parallel circumstances of contained activities in which expertise, experience, and credibility were significant factors, in which an outside consulting group with those characteristics was available (and preferably was familiar with the corporate environment and situation), and in which the corporate strategy is based upon retaining in house generalists to oversee and direct outsourced specialists for high defined tasks, one could reasonably expect the 30% cost containment estimate to be maintained.

ESTIMATED SAVINGS

Direct: $12,600

Indirect: efficient use of In-house generalists and outsourced experts

NOTES

It is unusal to be able to estimate direct cost savings with as precise reliability as in this case. Beause SueAnne was performing essentially the identifical tasks during the time period of the supply change analysis when she was both an in-house employee and an outsource consultant, the direct expenses associated with her employee salary and benefits and with her subsequent consultant fee are easily compared.

Not all outsourced positions result in indirect savings. Most companies justify the use of outsourcing on the basis of indirect savings: workforce flexibility, benefit expenses, short duration needs, and so on. In the regulatory compliance arena, these indirect savings may acrue, but the environment is unique in its reliance upon expertise and experience and upon the relationship and reputation of specific experts with key regulatory authorities. When a credible individual—in-house or outside consultant—testifies to compliance in accordance with the rules and guidelines of Federal Expert Witnesses, regulatory investigators (themselves generalists) are likely to accept that testimony with minimal confirmation.

Many organizations find credible experts highly valuable, but they need relatively contained activities and projects. The result is a real value in the use of outsourced consultants.

Case Code: B2A

Case: Blood Processor Audit System

Author: Weinberg

Industry: [X] Pharma   [ ] Biologics   [ ] Medical Device

Strategy: [ ] Requirements   [X] Audits   [ ] Quality by Design

              [ ] Outsource   [ ] Electronic Submissions   [ ] EMEA Overlap

BACKGROUND

A not-for-profit blood processor—accepting, testing, and packaging for transfusion human blood products—relies heavily on a computerized system for quality and safety controls. The FDA has conducted a series of field visits and has expressed strong skepticism about the reliability of the system. In order to assure product quality and to meet regulatory demands, the organization has decided to institute an auditing process aimed at monitoring the functionality and use of the computer system.

The software controlling the blood process procedures consists of 10 "soft" switches, initially set to "reject." As the blood sample is subject to different tests— HIV, HEPA, HEPB, HEPC, and so on—each switch is changed to "pass" if the results fall within positive and acceptable norms. At the end of the testing, if all switches are set at "accept," the blood is labeled as suitable for human use. If any of the switches remains at "reject," the blood is redirected for destruction or nonhuman applications (for testing for feline leukemia, for example).

From the time the original blood sample is drawn into one or more bags for processing and two test tubes (one for testing, one for archive), all labeled with an identical identification number, the entire procedure is automated. Safety and use decisions are made by computer without human intervention; labels are generated without human review. A system software error could conceivably (and historically has) result in a mislabeled blood bag, with serious potential human health implications.

Regulatory visits have highlighted outdated SOPs, inappropriate procedures, undocumented software changes and updates, untested code applications, and other evidence of inadequate validation and control.

STRATEGIC ACTION

The organization identified 24 blood processing sites scattered around the United States. Since their plan called for annual visits (24 audits per year) with the audit lasting one to two weeks, with audit teams traveling 50% of the time and located at a headquarters site half the time (to edit reports, update skills, provide training, etc.), two different audit teams were required. Each team would perform one audit per month, with teams switching audit lists annually so that each site would be audited by each team every two years.

Two three-person audit teams were established and trained, each consisting of an expert in computer systems operations and management, in documentation and quality control, and in regulatory affairs. A comprehensive checklist with more than 100 questions and control points was developed for use by the teams and by the management at the blood processing centers.

Once the two audit teams were thoroughly trained, a four-day training course for selected processing center staff was developed and presented. The plan was to make certain that everyone in the organization—field managers, auditors, and executives—was operating on the same page, with the same set of internal standards and the same definitions of control and validation.

After launch, the audits were conducted in random order, without advance notice to the processing sites. Each audit concluded with a verbal debriefing, followed within a week with a written report summary. If warranted, a repeat audit was scheduled after the site had an opportunity to correct deficiencies.

After the first four audits (two from each team) were completed, the audit teams met to assess the program and tweak the standards. Clarifications and modifications were communicated to the site staffs. The head of the audit teams then met informally with an FDA representative to communicate the details of the audit plan and to discuss suggestions.

In effect, this organization effectively assumed responsibility for self-regulation through a series of in depth site audits. The primary regulatory body responsibility shifted from the FDA to the audit group, with the FDA assuming the roles of advisor and of "reviewer of findings."

The cost of the program includes six full-time salaries ($145,000 per annum), a one-time consulting fee for the development of the standards and follow-up training ($35,000), and travel expenses.

In return, the organization shifted from a heavily regulated operation closely overseen by a very skeptical FDA with resulting product recalls, negative publicity, potential fines, legal liability, and so on, to a positive example of self-regulation with fewer product problems and significantly lower legal exposure.

EFFECT

The effects here are largely indirect. First, the organization has emerged as an industry leader in quality control, reversing an image and trend that was negatively affecting blood donations and other operations of the organization. The quality standards outlined in the checklist have become functional standards for all blood processors, and they are now routinely used by the FDA in conducting investigations of other sites as well as in reviewing the internal audit program in the case organization. By taking a proactive stand supporting quality control, the organization has demonstrated effective self-regulation, the proper and appropriate role of the FDA, and its own commitment to safety.

Second, the financial savings, while indirect, have been significant. At the advice of in-house attorneys, the organizations self-insurance product liability pool has been reduced by $5 million. This presumed savings is a result of the implementation of an effective auditing plan, the enthusiastic acceptance of that plan by the FDA, the resulting reduction in processing errors, and the favorable publicity the operation has generated.

Third, the organization gained a marketing advantage (or avoided a negative marketing disaster) through the generation of a positive quality control image, resulting largely from industry praise of the leadership position taken in quality. The specter of negative publicity resulting from medical problems traced to inaccurate blood testing has been replaced with a positive picture of an organization that has exceeded FDA requirements to institute their own system of regular audits and self-regulatory controls.

PROBLEMS/CHALLENGES

The biggest problem is the project's own success. As the FDA saw the effectiveness of the program, they first began to de facto require the same level of control in other blood processing organizations. Although organizations responded by adopting similar audit programs, the competitive advantage was diminished.

In addition, the FDA realized the vulnerability of blood processors to software problems in the approval decision systems employed. The FDA therefore declared those programs "medical devices" and launched a campaign requiring that the vendors of those software packages register their products under the 510(k) regulatory requirement. As vendors are complying, the relative value of the audit program is somewhat reduced (though the audits still effectively focus on and improve the quality of the use of the software and the quality assurances that surround its applications).

COST CONTAINMENT

This regulatory strategy required investment: a one-time consulting fee for the development of comprehensive standards; an ongoing department of two audit teams; and related travel expenses. Cost containment focused on (a) reduction of liability for production labeling errors, potentially resulting in utilization of a contaminated blood pack, and (b) the resulting FDA regulatory fines and expenses.

By implementing its own auditing strategy, the organization effectively increased its quality control to the level exceeding industry standards and FDA requirements, reducing its liability significantly. In addition, by assuming a self-regulation role, the expenses associated with unexpected and crisis control surrounding an FDA investigational visit were rationalized and normalized with a continuous regulatory oversight providing ongoing evidence of high levels of quality assurance and control.

ESTIMATED SAVINGS

Direct: $5 million (liability reserve)

Indirect: positive image enhancement

NOTES

The decision of the FDA to treat software used in the blood processing industry as a medical device subject to the 510(k) registration requirements proved both popular and controversial. Software vendors, learning of the liability protection and marketing advantage that could acrue from and FDA "stamp of approval," have been patiently awaiting the extension of the concept to other software categories (despite numerous FDA hints, there is no current program to permit registration of LIMS, MES, or other software). The industry embraced the idea of FDA approval of the validation and quality control of the software so critical to operations. The political and general public, however, criticized the move as removing some performance responsibility from the licensed product distributor, a fundamental FDA principle. Perhaps that controversy is the reason the program has not been extended to other software.

While image is difficult to define and all but impossible to quantify, it can be a very important organizational asset, very difficult and expensive to build and to repair. The organization forming the basis of this (composite) case depends on funding in part from its blood processing business and in part from public donations; the second income source is particularly vulnerable to image issues. A reputation for poor quality control, or even for the necessity for tight external FDA oversight, could have significant impact, hence further justifying the self-regulatory audit strategy described here.

Case Code: P1O

Case: Metabolic Pharma SOPs

Author: Weinberg

Industry: [X] Pharma   [ ] Biologics   [ ] Medical Device

Strategy: [ ] Requirements   [ ] Audits   [ ] Quality by Design

               [X] Outsource   [ ] Electronic Submissions   [ ] EMEA Overlap

BACKGROUND

Metabolic Pharma, Inc. is a Florida-based virtual drug development company. The newly formed organization licenses conduct clinical tests and brings to market pharmaceutical products designed to treat orphan metabolic diseases. The company consists of a President (Mark), a VP-Medical Director (Melissa), a VP-Regulatory/ QA Director (Robert), and an Administrative Assistant (Martha). Once President Mark identifies and licenses a promising molecule, VP Melissa designs the clinical studies and contracts with a Contract Research Organization (CRO) while VP Robert submits the appropriate Investigatory New Drug Application (IND) to the FDA.

After three months of operation, Regulatory VP Robert realized that the company needed to develop and operate under a series of Standard Operating Procedures in order to be compliant with FDA regulations. He developed two plans:

Plan A. Hire a full-time Quality/Technical Writer professional to develop the approximately 12 SOPs required, estimated to require two years for analysis, development, revision, final wording, and implementation (about one SOP per month). Cost: $120,000 salary plus 30% overhead, $156,000, times two years: $312,000.

Plan B. Outsource the SOP development by purchasing a "standard set" of SOPs ($5000) and hiring a technical writer for three months ($30,000) to revise them over a three-month period (each of the company employees to assume responsibility for three SOPs, one per month, to review and edit. The tech writer is to incorporate recommended changes into final version. Total Cost: $35,000 (plus some executive time in review of SOPs, presumably fit into planning downtime).

Note that Plan B achieves compliance in three months rather than two years.

STRATEGIC ACTION

While short-term cost containment is a significant goal of the Metabolic Pharma organization, two other long-term financial issues are relevant to decision-making. First, the organization's success is pinned to efficiency and speed to market. Please orphan products have relatively small markets, profitability flows from FDA protections against competition and from the protections offered from patents. Both of these protections have limited durations, and delays (caused by regulatory or other factors) can be expensive in the long run. The company cannot afford to operate for two years without appropriate SOPs, risking clinical holds in the future.

The second problem is more subtle. In virtual companies, there is a tendency toward "headcount creep." While the goal is to outsource as much a possible, there is a continuous pressure to add people to the payroll when they are working on relatively long-term projects, and a hesitation to terminate them at project termination when that individual has (a) performed successfully, (b)forged relationships with other employees, and (c) can be productive in the future. A person joining the staff for two years is likely to become a permanent employee, making real contributions at the end of that period but increasing the headcount. If the company wants to truly remain virtual, it must fight this "creep" tendency on every front.

These two factors, coupled with the financial savings from the outsource strategy and reinforced by the organizations "virtual" philosophy encouraging outsourcing wherever possible, makes the strategic decision an easy one.

The Metabolic Pharmaceutical company assigned Robert, VP of Regulatory, the SOP responsibility, Robert first made a list, with input from all four employees, of the 12 SOPs needed. He then found a web-based organization that would sell a template of these 12 topic SOPs for a fee of approximately $5000. Robert then divided the list into four categories and gave three SOP templates to each of the four employees with instructions to "review, revise, and edit" over the next four weeks. During those four weeks, Robert contracted with a technical writer: This person was given the 12 edited SOPs with revisions and was assigned the task of producing 12 "penultimate" SOPs over the course of the next 90 days.

When the technical writer delivered the "penultimate drafts," they were copied and distributed to all four employees, who were given a week to read and comment. Robert then collected the comments, made any necessary revisions, and distributed the now final copies for signature and implementation.

The entire process was completed in under three months at a cost of less than $35,000. While additional SOPs may well be required over time, this process provided Metabolic Pharma with a basic set of procedures rapidly, efficiently, inexpensively, and without adding headcount to the company.

EFFECT

Metabolic Pharma, Inc. managed to meet all of its long- and short-term goals. Achieving short-term cost containment, the company saved approximately $275,000 in the development of the required 12 basic Standard Operating Procedures.

On a longer-term cost-containment horizon, the company avoided regulatory delays and adverse findings by having all 12 SOPs in place prior to the submission of its first IND and initial clinical study (the clinical study itself, of course, was conducted under the SOPs of the selected CRO). This appropriate sequencing prevented potential loss of patent and orphan protection time, increasing long-term value of the organization.

And by avoiding adding a two-year employee to the team for SOP development and future documentation needs, the company delayed the (seemingly inevitable) headcount creep that affects so many virtual organizations. A three-month technical writer, operating out of her own home office and visiting the company an average of twice a week, did not become a permanent fixture: Though she is likely to used on an outsource basis on future projects, there are no pressures to offer her a permanent position; she remained an adjunct to, not a member of the company team.

These three advantages of outsourcing make the option very attractive, though in many cases the initial cost of the outsource operation may be a greater expense, with savings accruing from the secondary indirect benefits. In this case, largely because of the outsource availability of pre-written SOP templates, all three outsourcing aspects were cost-effective.

PROBLEMS/CHALLENGES

The most significant challenge in this case is the limitation of number and detail of the Standard Operating Procedures development. Many companies write such extremely detailed SOPs and generate so many different SOPs, that it is all but impossible for employees to know and understand them all. Since a real regulatory concern is the question of whether or not an organization is following its SOPs, the result is many unnecessary adverse findings. A new company like Metabolic Pharma has the advantage of avoiding a historical backlog of unneeded SOPs and can focus on the few major necessary topics with sufficient detail to provide guidance for employees.

The other, much more minor challenge facing Metabolic was how to force executives with busy schedules to conform to firm deadlines. Two tactics were used;

first, the company agreed to a default result: If you failed to provide feedback, the SOP was considered acceptable. Only by meeting the deadline did you have a chance for input. Anyone late in giving their feedback bought everyone else lunch until they caught up!

COST CONTAINMENT

The Metabolic Pharma company made use of outsourcing for the development of Standard Operating Procedures by first purchasing a set of SOP templates, and then using an (outsourced) technical writing to revise those SOPs to the customized needs of the company.

By not developing the basic SOPs "from scratch," the company saved initial expenses but more importantly avoided an increase in number of full-time employees ("headcount creep") and sped the process to assure regulatory compliance in advance of regulatory submissions and first studies.

The result was an efficient three-month project that provided an appropriate and accurate set of basic operating procedures for the company without lengthy delays, multiple revisions, or overly complex final SOPs.

ESTIMATED SAVINGS

Direct: $277,000

Indirect: speed; low headcount

NOTES

The quality of available SOP templates varies widely: Reputable companies will provide a listing of SOPs available, along with a sample of any SOP of your choice. Those labeled "templates"—identifying issues and procedures but not attempting to be "fill in the blanks"—are generally the more useful and sophisticated. Recommendation: Use the templates as assisting tools rather than as SOPs to be adopted as is.

"Headcount creep" is a problem in all companies, particularly in start-ups attempting to operate as virtual companies. Once good people are brought on board, they prove themselves as valuable and make real contributions beyond the limits of their initial projects. If headcount isn't an issue, this is a fine method of growth. But if business plans, investors, and other pressures force low head count, it creates a real dilemma. No one wants to fire a valued employee: Its bad for morale, it has serious financial implications (particularly in Europe), and there are important ethical issues. Outsourcing, when used effectively, represents a reasoned response as long as it is used to have individuals with specific skills available for finite projects. If your outsourced consultants are beginning to win longevity awards, it's time to reconsider the policy: You may simply be paying an unnecessary management fee for what are de facto full-time employees.

Case Code: P2Q

Case: Pharmaceutical Manufacturing Pilot

Author: Weinberg

Industry: [X] Pharma   [ ] Biologics   [ ] Medical Device

Strategy: [ ] Requirements   [ ] Audits   [X] Quality by Design

              [ ] Outsource   [ ] Electronic Submissions   [ ] EMEA Overlap

BACKGROUND

The company is a large international pharmaceutical manufacturing organization located in Eastern Pennsylvania. As a part of the process of developing a strong in-house understanding of the Quality by Design concept, the company has formed a task force to pilot the use of QbD on a basic pharmaceutical manufacturing line.

The pilot team is headed by Charles, a senior manufacturing engineer, and includes representatives from Quality Assurance (Terri), Regulatory (Anita), and CMC (Sam). They have chosen a tablet line that mixes active pharmaceutical ingredients (API) and substrates, presses the mixture in a tablet press, coats the tablet, stencils the company logo on each tablet, packages in bubble packs, adds labeling information, and boxes for shipment.

The team began their task by conducting a Risk Analysis to identify the key control points in the manufacturing process, including appropriate mix of materials, proper humidity and pressure in the tablet press, complete sugar coating of each tablet, proper stenciling, package seals, and so on. Once these control points are specified, a Design Space analysis was used to define acceptable performance ranges for each measurement. Finally, the manufacturing line was redesigned using Process Analytical Technology concepts to include (a) sensors, set to the design space specifications, at each control point, and (b) cybernetic adjustors to tweak the process (wherever possible) to near instantly readjust any control points out of design space specification. These three tasks together consumed approximately three months, the majority of the time spent on the process analytical technology steps.

When the pilot project was operational, the team measured productivity, quality, and other measures and compared the results with those of traditional manufacturing lines.

STRATEGIC ACTION

The team modified a manufacturing production line designed to bubble-pack and box coated tablets to incorporate the three key principles of Quality by Design (Risk Assessment, Design Space, and Process Analytical Technology). The result was a functioning pilot operation with clearly identified control points; defined ranges of acceptability for each control point; and frequent, self-correcting measurements for those control point ranges.

The team was able to compare the pre-QbD (no qa/qc) and post-Qbd production, along with the parallel production on a similar but non-QbD production line (traditional qa/qc) , according to three dimensions:

Production volume/hour

Quality volume (number of units passing QA and QC checks)

Operating cost per tablet

	No QA/QC	QbD	Trad QA/QC
Volume	80,000	78,000	79,000
QA Vol	—	77,000	76,000
Cost	$0.030	$0.034	$0.038

Note that it is reasonable to interpret the "no QA/QC" column—that is, without any controls and hence without any opportunity to find and reject mismanufactured tablets—as the definition of optimum productivity on these pilot manufacturing lines, combined with minimal possible cost. These are, of course, false norms since they measure all tablets produced rather than all acceptable tablets produced.

There is, then, a potential $0.4 cent per tablet saving to be realized in this model by using QbD over traditional QA/QC inspection and control methods. This seemingly small saving per tablet can be significant in a factory producing millions of tablets per week, assuming that the post of QbD implementation does not offset the lowered production cost. But how is this manufacturing and quality constant containment related to regulatory cost containment?

Representing the team, Charles presented the tentative findings at a major national conference, and he sought feedback from the FDA. The response took the form of three general (nonbinding) observations:

- Once the presence of an effective QbD system was established, the need for frequent FDA visits was significantly reduced.
- With a QbD system in place, the likelihood of a product recall (or destruction order) was significantly reduced.
- Under a QbD system, production system modification notifications would be rapidly accepted and (with the Design Space) less frequently needed.

Based upon these general assurances, the pilot team estimated that an annual savings (resulting from reduced regulatory time, fewer recalls, etc.) would average about $250,000. They estimated that the cost of QbD installation approximated $500,000 (initial investment), providing a two-year payback with significant cost containment in the third and subsequent years of operation.

EFFECT

The Quality by Design (QbD) construct should have a significant impact on regulatory costs, directly through the automation of the quality assurance and control process. To the extent that the Regulatory role is to interpret FDA agency standards, requirements, and guidelines to the industry, the analysis and interpretation of the QbD moving target will largely be a regulatory responsibility. And to the extent that the other major Regulatory role is the representation of the quality processes to the agency, QbD provides the framework and methodology for demonstrating that compliance.

While QbD is yet to be fully defined, its evolutionary path is now clear. In its most skeletal form, QbD will involve some sort of risk assessment, some design space analysis to define the acceptable ranges within that risk level, and a Process Analytical technology approach to establishing continuous (or frequent) process monitoring for deviations from the design space defined range, along with cybernetic correction of those deviations.

This pilot experiment, adding to the body of experience, is a case (composite from several similar experiments) providing an example of how QbD could potentially contain some production costs and some of the regulatory costs associated with that production monitoring. Particularly in a linear tablet mix–press–coat–package process the comparative QbD advantages are relatively easy to estimate.

There is little question about whether or not QbD will improve quality monitoring Spot checks and quarantine retests are better accomplished with continuous conformity monitoring. Replacing as it does spot checks and quarantine retests will on the spot, continuous conformity monitoring. Whether nor not that improvement justifies cost is still moot, but showing promise.

PROBLEMS/CHALLENGES

The two greatest challenges here are obtaining a clear definition of the "moving target" that is Quality by Design, as well as obtaining from the Food and Drug Administration a clear commitment to appropriately limited regulatory oversight once a QbD system has been installed. If the FDA is able to review and accept the QbD system has an effective control of the now automated QA/QC process, a great deal of the uncertainty of FDA visits would be eliminated. Other than initial approval of the QbD controls, as well as occasional reviews of Standard Operation Procedures and documentation, a facility would be truly self-regulated. Such a situation would also provide the agency with a rational method of focusing its underfunded resources on areas of greatest concern, including un-QbD monitored facilities. Just as the GMPs provided the FDA with a chance to step back from primary regulator to overseer of internal QA/QC operations, an established QbD standard and registration would allow the agency to delegate direct oversight to automated systems and concentrate resources in areas of greatest vulnerability.

COST CONTAINMENT

Charles' team explored the possibility of utilizing a Quality by Design (QbD) approach to the automation of quality assurance and control in a pilot manufacturing process. The result was a clear demonstration of controlling quality costs, and hence containing regulatory costs, in this simplified tablet mix–press–coat–package process. Because the FDA has offered QbD as a regulatory enhancement, tentatively promising to reduce oversight, speed reviews of production changes, and generally ease regulatory burdens, quality investments herein directly translate to regulatory cost control.

As QbD is fine-tuned and FDA general promises gel into actual policies, the implementation of automated quality assurance and control systems should significantly reduce regulatory compliance expenses by providing greater latitude to companies to self-regulate once the FDA has audited and reviewed QbD systems in situo.

ESTIMATED SAVINGS

Direct: $1,250,000 over five years

Indirect: FDA acceptance of increased self-regulation responsibility

NOTES

This case is based upon a work in progress—QbD—and both anticipates and sets the stage for expected FDA developments in automated quality control and assurance. The three QbD steps discussed—risk analysis, design space, and process analytical technology—currently define the construct, but what if any additional dimensions might be added is still very much in doubt. The goal of QbD is to increase the self-regulation of the regulated company, and hence decrease the direct FDA involvement in operations. This shift of balance is expected to produce cost-containment benefits, particularly as it speeds the process of making production line modifications and control level adjustments. In theory a QbD operation should eventually reduce headcount in both the Quality and Regulatory departments, though it is expected that such savings may be delayed until QbD is well established and well demonstrated.

While QbD—defined by the three dimensions discussed above—will significantly automate the quality process, it should be noted that just one of those dimensions can account for the majority of the increased control and decreased cost. Process Analytical Technology, already in place in many organizations, provides the continuous cybernetic monitoring and often is a bonus capability of remote monitoring. While Risk Assessment and Design Space further refine and justify the PAT control levels, PAT alone can make significant inroads toward self-regulation.

Case Code: D1Q

Case: Quality By Design in A Blood Analysis Device

Author: Weinberg

Industry: [ ] Pharma   [ ] Biologics   [X] Medical Device

Strategy: [ ] Requirements   [ ] Audits   [X] Quality by Design
              [ ] Outsource   [ ] Electronic Submissions   [ ] EMEA Overlap

BACKGROUND

A global medical instrument and device company headquartered in the EMEA (Netherlands) has developed a free-standing robotic blood analyzer primarily aimed at the US market. The device has complex software and hardware designed to move specially designed test tubes of human blood through a series of plated test stations, using internally stored reagents to perform a variety of analytical tests. The user selects the appropriate tests from a menu, tracks the original test tube, and receives test results in both raw data and analyzed results forms (displayed on a screen and directed to a connected printer).

The device has been designed with three QbD concepts utilized to maintain accuracy of results and interpretations. First, design engineers and quality control personnel performed a detailed risk analysis to determine critical control points in the sample tracking system, the robotic manipulation system, each testing system, the analyses systems, and the reporting system. Second, the design team used a Design Space analysis to determine the acceptable parameter ranges for each identified critical point variable. This process included physical measurements of the robotic test tube manipulation chain, the dispensing quantity measurement system, the reagent dispensing system, the plate geographic system, the result measurement systems, and the analytical systems (including statistical interpretation ranges). Finally the team installed process analytical control devices at all critical points, set to measure the ranges determined, with cybernetic corrective capability as well as problem signal capabilities. Together, this QbD approach provided automated internal quality control and assurance capacity.

In the 510(k) medical device submission the organization specified period calibration controls and testing of the QbD system as appropriate quality assurance procedures, and it provided evidence that the device did not require additional oversight to assure continued accuracy and reliability.

STRATEGIC ACTION

The organization has determined that the ultimate value of the product and position in its niche is based upon the self-contained nature of the device. It can command a high price point and establish a significant competitive advantage by position itself as fully automated, requiring no expert human intervention. Coupled with rugged construction, this makes the blood analyzer ideal for field use in potential combat, disaster, and other nonlaboratory environments.

The one vulnerability or exception to complete automation is quality control. Similar devices require constant monitoring, quality checking, and expert oversight that significantly limits its field value. By employing the principles and practical procedures of QbD, however, the company has overcome this barrier: It has automated the routine quality control and assurance functions just as it has automated testing and analysis.

Calculation of the savings produced by the use of this automated regulatory compliance process is problematic. By its nature and intentional application, QbD is fully integrated into the device design, resulting in little real increase in component parts (one engineer estimated that the increase in sensors and software controls represented a per unit cost of about $3.00, less than 1% of the overall production cost). Of course, design costs, difficult to estimate, probably run much higher.

The automated nature of the qa.qc process provided a unique (at last for a while) niche for the device increasing its value and hence its price and profitability. Similar devices without QbD capability are marketed at a price point approximately 24% lower than this blood analyzer (though there are some key testing and analytical differences), a per unit figure of about $1152 per device sold. Assuming the same or equivalent engineering and production costs, this represents a profit differential of approximately $1150 per unit: In the first year of sales the increased profit would therefore be an aggregate $1,444,000.

Skepticism over any attempt to attribute such a figure solely to cost containment of regulatory compliance is highly appropriate. Clearly a unit that has in effect "built-in" compliance has a market advantage, but the measurement of that advantage is inexact and to assume that such an advantage directly translates to increased valuation in selling price is problematic at best.

An alternative (but equally flawed) calculation of regulatory savings can be derived through an estimate of the cost of human quality assurance (monthly testing and monitoring of the system): 12 person days @$500 per day + $150 overhead = $650/day * 12 days = $7800 per year, estimating a five-year depreciation totals $39,000 in regulatory review costs per device. If the value differential of the similar device without QbD represents a decreased cost of $1150, the per unit value (cost containment) of automate regulatory functions is estimated as $37,850. Again, it is a highly problematic figure. It is clear that as QbD becomes a norm for automating compliance, new and better methods of calculating savings will be needed.

EFFECT

The effect of utilizing the principles and concepts of Quality by Design (QbD) in a medical device (in this case, a blood analyzer) is the practical automation of quality assurance and control. While regular calibration and spot checks are still recommended, the QbD process provides continuous monitoring and cybernetic correction of all critical points whenever the values of those points fall outside of defined design space limits. Because the initial 510(k) submission of the device is reviewed by the FDA and (presumably) approved prior to marketing, with or without supplemental Pre-market Approval (PMA) data, the FDA in effect provides a prior approval of the qa process. The system therefore has an implied endorsement of regulatory acceptance of control and of resulting data and analysis.

Savings and regulatory cost containment are not only accrued by the medical device designer and manufacturer: Users of the system to analyze blood results for use in clinical trials or other applications will enjoy significant containment in regulatory expenses since the device has preapproved built-in quality controls. FDA approval of the system in effect says that the data outcomes meet regulatory standards as long as the application environment follows specifications and normally accepted practices (SOPs).

While QbD was originally intended for use in pharmaceutical manufacturing, this extension of the process meets the spirit of the initiative, providing cost controls without sacrificing quality controls. The FDA is in effect reviewing the automated process of overseeing quality and, finding that acceptable, endorsing the end result of the application. The case, and the expansion of the QbD initiative it represents, can serve as a harbinger for a new approach to regulatory oversight that offers significant advantages in both cost containment and quality.

PROBLEMS/CHALLENGES

The FDA QbD initiative is in its earliest stages of evolution and will no doubt be modified over time. Currently the approach has three elements: risk assessment, design space analysis, and continuous and cybernetic process analytical technology monitoring. While not applicable for all situations, this automation of the quality control process represents a significant cost-containment strategy for medical devices and well as other areas.

Other than the fluid nature of the QbD definitions, the major problem encountered in this case derives from the nature of reagent testing. Distorted or false results will be obtained if the reagent utilized is outdated, contaminated, or otherwise inappropriate. The QbD controls will not detect these problems, resulting in (a) a continuing need to calibrate and inspect the apparatus between applications and (b) a continuing need to test new reagent for purity and activity before accepting a new infusion into the device.

COST CONTAINMENT

Calculation of the indirect savings—resulting from prior regulatory approval of the analysis device potentially utilized in clinical studies and other applications—is very difficult to calculate accurately. Biannual validation and quarterly quality testing of application results by an outside contract is estimated at $30,000; that cost is effectively eliminated, while the calibration and inspection expenses are retained.

Direct cost containment for the original equipment manufacturer is roughly estimated at $1,440,000 (for the total number of units sold).

Both of these figures should be viewed skeptically: There clearly is a savings accrued from the QbD automation of quality control, realized by both the OEM and the end user, quantifying that savings is more magic than science.

ESTIMATED SAVINGS

Direct: perhaps $1,440,000

Indirect: $30,000 per unit utilized in a regulated environment

NOTES

Quality by Design (QbD) is very much as work in progress: To date, this is the first application of QbD to a medical device and is the first attempt to use a QbD device for clinical testing applications as with the blood analyzer. Several pharmaceutical manufacturing QbD trials are underway, and no doubt will result in some modification and maturation of the QbD concepts, potentially necessitating some changes in the device described in this case (and subsequent re-review of the device by the FDA). Experience suggests, however, that most conceptual changes will tend toward reducing rather than adding to the regulatory burden: QbD is likely to be a less rigorous rather than a more extensive guideline.

The classification of testing systems like this blood analyzer as a medical device is not a universal concept, and it is probably not necessary to register such equipment under the 510(k) provision. There are distinct marketing advantages in such a registration, however, and FDA guidelines for blood processing and testing make this special category of equipment somewhat of a gray area. In this case the analyzer was accepted as a medical device, was reviewed against QbD emerging standards, and was found to be in compliance with validation and quality standards through the effective automation of the quality control and quality assurance processes.

Case Code: P1R

Case: Manufacturing Formulation System

Author: Weinberg

Industry: [X] Pharma   [ ] Biologics   [ ] Medical Device

Strategy: [X] Requirements   [ ] Audits   [ ] Quality by Design

[ ] Outsource   [ ] Electronic Submissions   [ ] EMEA Overlap

BACKGROUND

This traditional large-molecule drug development, manufacturing, and distribution company is located in Eastern Pennsylvania. The case focuses on a division of merged company, combining two of the largest and oldest pharmaceutical firms in the United States. The case focuses on a manufacturing facility in which two active ingredients are combined with an inert substrate into a tablet, which is then packaged and labeled for over-the-counter (OTC) sales in Europe, South American, and Asia and for both ethical drug and OTC use (depending on tablet strength) in the United States. The product is used for symptomatic control of common chronic condition.

The facility is governed by a set of more than 400 complex and detailed standard operating procedures that have evolved over a 30-year period. Little or no attempt has been made to update, screen, or even review these standard operating procedures (SOPs). On an annual basis (usually during the post-holiday lull) the division President and VP for Quality sign each SOP coversheet, approving the set for continued use: All 400+ procedures are signed at once, generally in a single morning; it is highly doubtful that either the President or Vice President actually read any of the SOPs.

Over the years the set of SOPs have been expanded (often without culling of outdated, obsolete, or contradictory earlier procedures) in response to new FDA interpretations, inspection comments, industry rumor, and the recommendations of outside consultants and internal executives. As a result, the set of SOPs—if followed—would call for a considerable collection of extra and obsolete compliance efforts.

A recent FDA visit cited the company for not following its SOPs—to do so would have been all but impossible, given their contradictory nature. The 483 finding did not mention, however, that the policies the company was following greatly exceeded regulatory requirements.

STRATEGIC ACTION

In response to the FDA's findings and internal realization of the complexity of the SOP set, the company began a three-step process. First, all SOPs were reviewed to eliminate outdated, contradictory, obsolete, and inappropriate standards. Second, the organization developed an "SOP on SOPs" policy designed to improve the review process, periodically police the SOP set, and assure the appropriateness of all SOPs in use. Finally, the company began a lengthy process of analysis of the actual operational definitions of all formal and informal requirements, focusing on (a) what is actually required and (b) where, when, and why the company intended to exceed those minimal standards.

The process of SOP review and revision took the internal Quality Assurance and Regulatory Department staff approximately nine months, but resulted in a much streamlined set of 46 (electronic) SOPs accessible to all employees and controlled (for update and revision) by a centralized process.

Simultaneously, the company developed and implemented a new policy of executive review, which passed responsibility for detailed analysis to an Assistant to the President (who then prepared a formal memo for the President's signature, indicating that the entire SOP set had been reviewed and approved), along with a review for conformity to approval procedures by the VP for Quality. This policy was developed in 45 days (overlapping the SOP review process) and is now implemented on an annual basis.

Finally, the company utilized a recently retired quality expert as a consultant to determine the operational definitions of relevant standards and requirements and to recommend specific revisions to the SOP set to conform to the minimum compliance requirements. The expert also indicated areas in which expansion beyond minimal requirements would have a direct and significant impact on quality. The VP of Quality also added recommendations for enhancement beyond minimum standards. This consultant review took six months, overlapping the SOP review and revision, and served as input into the final stage of that review process.

Expenses related to the project included:

In-house efforts in SOP revision: two people @ $80,000 + 30% overhead

9/12 of the year: $156,000

In-house executive time, total of 12 days @ $200,000 + 30% overhead $46,800

Six-month fixed price consulting project: $120,000

SUBTOTAL: $322,800

Savings, directly calculated as reduction-in-force of three QA persons managing, updating, enforcing, and training SOP system @ 65,000 + 30%: $253,500

Indirect: avoidance of FDA 483 criticism (possible fines, short-term effect on stock price, disruption of manufacturing, short-term effect on product market value): $3,500,000

TOTAL: $3,753,500 − 322,800 = $3,430,700 (see NOTES)

EFFECT

By updating the SOP set, the company increased the likelihood of compliance with those procedures and gained the opportunity to modify or eliminate requirements that significantly exceed actual regulatory standards. Examples include reducing number of tested API samples from arbitrary to appropriate numbers, eliminating redundant checks on humidity recently made unnecessary by improved automated monitoring technology, and excessive and nonrequired inventory software testing controlled instead through the use of independently validated and tested commercial computer software.

The effects of these improvements are not only production cost controls but also additional quality confidence because (a) workers can rely upon the Standard Operating Procedures as guidance and training documents, (b) Qa and QC professionals have reasonable standards of measurement and control, and (c) regulatory affairs professionals can demonstrate competence and compliance to FDA investigators.

The case also eliminated or minimized the potentiality for future adverse effects, including but not limited to (a) adverse publicity after an FDA adverse finding (or more serious action), affecting stock price, consumer confidence, fines, and possible recall expenses, (b) a loss of FDA confidence in the operation, (c) increasing frequency of future visits and potentially delaying future approvals, and (d) the possibility through poor quality control of a product contamination or toxicity problem.

More directly, FDA policy calls for holding companies to the standards established in their own SOPs: Complex, contradictory, and excessive SOPs result in increased compliance expense.

PROBLEMS/CHALLENGES

The most significant challenge faced by the organization in this case was the determination of actual industry standards and regulatory expectations of quality controls and appropriate testing standards. The company here was fortunate to find an individual with a combination of extensive industry experience and strong regulatory contacts. Without access to an experienced consultant or in house regulatory compliance and CMC expert, those "real" standards are very difficult to determine. One estimate suggests that most US-based manufacturing facilities exceed minimal standards by factors in excess of 50%; while no doubt some of that excess is a result of conscious decisions based upon unusual quality situations, it is likely that a good deal of that additional effort is "insurance" attempts to maintain compliance in the absence of clear standards. The challenge might be better met if organizations would determine independently appropriate and justifiable standards; document those justifications, and provide the FDA with the rationales independent of attempts to read between the regulatory lines.

COST CONTAINMENT

In this case the company realized some savings in reducing the headcount necessary to maintain an unnecessarily complex and convoluted set of SOPs, and (it) invested in a clear and reduced definitional standard set to avoid potential future expenses flowing form poor quality control, lack of compliance (as employees were held to the inadequate standards), and unnecessarily high and confusing quality control standards resulting from a lack of clear definitions of necessary controls and regulatory requirements.

Although the savings resulting from this avoidance of future expense is difficult to quantify and specify, top management was and remains convinced that they had "dodged a bullet" in avoiding a scenario of extensive regulatory criticism and escalating controls and restrictions. While estimates of the value of that avoidance are problematic at best, it is clear that the strategy adopted was considered more than financially justified.

ESTIMATED SAVINGS

Direct: See NOTES
Indirect: $3,430,700

NOTES

This organization's estimate of savings as a result of the operational definition compliance strategy is highly problematic. When asked to calculate the future cost avoidance afforded by a much improved SOP system that minimized extraneous controls and improved regulatory acceptance, top management named a figure of $3.5 million and then worked backward to a justification of estimate. Perhaps in this case it is safe to conclude that savings are likely to greatly exceed expenditure in the implementation of the strategy, but signficant skepticism should be attached to any exact or even rounded estimate of the amount of that saving.

It is important to note that the actual savings in this case came from two major changes: (a) the reorganization and updating of the SOP set and (b) the revision of that set in response to a clear understanding of actual definitions of appropriate levels of quality control, quality assurance, and testing. The first change made the second one possible: It is the strategy of establishing clear operational definitions of actual requirements and guidelines that results in ongoing and signficant cost containment. In this case, a poorly written and managed set of SOPs necessitated revision; in many organizations those SOPs are modern, well-designed, and well-maintained, but contain standards based upon vague requirements that hold organizations to procedures well in excess of any real benefit for compliance necessity.

Case Code: D2R

Case: Plastic condoms

Author: Weinberg

Industry: [ ] Pharma   [ ] Biologics   [X] Medical Device

Strategy: [X] Requirements   [ ] Audits   [ ] Quality by Design

[ ] Outsource   [ ] Electronic Submissions   [ ] EMEA Overlap

BACKGROUND

Latex and latex-derivative condoms are manufactured using a relatively simple process of dipping a steel shaft in the liquefied rubber-like material. The FDA requires two tests of the final product: The first, used on every condom, is a spark applied to the steel shaft once it is covered; if the spark makes contact, the condom has a gap or hole, and it is rejected (hence the "pretested" label that may cause some high-schoolers to snicker). The nonrejected devices are rolled off the shaft and prepared for packaging; a random sample is subjected to the second, more rigorous test: Water is injected into the condom to determine whether or not it maintains integrity under pressure. If the sample passes, the batch is packaged, labeled, and distributed (the actual tested condoms are destroyed).

A British company developed an alternate device made of plastic rather than a latex-like material. This plastic design has certain product advantages, particularly in protection against HIV and other sexually transmitted diseases. But the manufacturing process, an injection mold design, is not suitable to the spark test. It is suitable to a nondestructive version of the water test, however; all produced condoms are subject to the more rigorous test. The result is that batches of these plastic condoms are all more thoroughly tested that are traditional condoms. The spirit and intent of the testing regulation is preserved (or excelled), but the letter of the requirement— the less effective spark test for all, the more reliable water test for a sample—is not followed.

In-house advisors informed management that, to assure compliance and FDA approval, the procedures must be modified to include a second testing of a sample of the produced condoms, even though this additional testing added significant expense and no useful information. While accepting that American bureaucratic procedures might require such a worthless step, the UK management team decided to investigate further and sought additional advice.

STRATEGIC ACTION

A regulatory consulting team visited the production site and developed a detailed description of the manufacturing and testing process; secured documentary evidence including test protocols and records, product failure and recall records, and quality control Standard Operating Procedures; and obtained and independently tested product samples.

With a complete evidentiary package demonstrating that the 100% water test protocol was equal or superior to the specified 100% spark test (an inferior test) and the random sample water test (performed on only on a small minority of the condoms traditionally produced), the team then developed a comprehensive testing plan document, intended to provide an operational definition of the qa/qc process and of compliance with applicable regulations and guidelines. A risk analysis, demonstrating the low-level danger to public health and safety, was added.

The team requested and met with a group of FDA representatives responsible for review of medical device applications, including an FDA "condom expert." The evidence of control was presented and explained: Other than clarification questions during the presentation, the FDA group had no comments or recommendations.

This complete evidentiary package was appended to the 510(k) application, with a detailed cover letter explaining how the process designed and employed provided greater quality assurance than that specified in the FDA guidance documents and clearly met the compliance definition.

The FDA approved the 510(k) as written and, at a subsequent visit to the production site, had no adverse findings or comments regarding the testing protocol. As newer and varying condom technologies emerge at other companies, the FDA has tacitly accepted the clarified definition of its testing requirements as, in effect, "providing testing security equivalent to the spark test and random sample water test."

The cost of the redundant second (sample) water test recommended by the in-house advisors would have added an estimated $2,200,000 per annum to the overall production of the plastic condoms. The comprehensive cost (not including nominal travel expenses) of the outside consulting team was a total of $72,000.

The direct cost containment of this clear definition strategy was $2,128,000 in the first year of product (the savings were slightly higher in other years, because the outside team's involvement was restricted to an annual review meeting to assure continued compliance, at a significantly reduced fee).

There was no indirect cost containment: All savings in this case were direct and reliably estimated.

EFFECT

There are two major effects of the development of a clear definition of the intent of the condom testing protocol—in effect, of the "industry standard" procedure. First, for the industry as a whole, the new definition of equivalency rather than exact conformity opened the door for new innovations in materials and technologies. The "female condom," for example, which utilizes a welded plastic technology, would have been unlikely to meet the inflexible standard, and new nonlatex materials would have required significantly more expensive testing to demonstrate compliance.

Second, for the specific condom company in question, the approach of clearly demonstrating control with effective documentation of well-designed procedures provided the opportunity to shift the regulatory question from the conservative and limiting "Does this device pass the preestablished tests?" to the more meaningful and appropriate question "Has the organization demonstrated quality assurance and control through testing *equivalent* to that provided in the preestablished tests?" In effect, the organization has developed its own clear, supported, and persuasive operational definition of the concept underlying the FDA guidance, and hence has demonstrated regulatory compliance with its own appropriate and logical variation.

Both effects are the result of a larger principle—that is, that the pharmaceutical, biologics, and device industries are self-regulated and that the job of the FDA is to assure that self-regulation. All too often the industry and the agency forget this principle and, because of intimidation, fear, or conservatism, avoid appropriate and superior procedures rather than "rock the boat." The FDA (on its best days) prefers that the company assumes responsibility for justifying its own definitions of compliance, and the public good often demands that affirmative action.

PROBLEMS/CHALLENGES

The problem underlying this case was intimidation. All too many in-house regulatory professionals and advisors are afraid of dealing with the FDA. They seem to opt for the path of unquestioning following of established norms, guidelines, and industry standards, convinced that any variation is likely to result in disaster.

The reality is that the persons in the FDA—concerned individually as is the general population with wanting to protect turf, to avoid being made a fool of; skeptical of an industry it is designed to oversee; and often concerned that they are forced to make decisions in excess of their own expertise—are generally dedicated individuals with strong altruistic motivations. A credible presentation of clear self-regulating controls is likely to be met with interest, appropriate scientific skepticism, and a spirit of cooperative inquiry. The challenge is to understand and then explain the intent of a requirement and to clearly and appropriately demonstrate compliance with that requirement.

COST CONTAINMENT

The cost-containment advantage in this case flowed directly from avoiding the necessity of conducting, on an ongoing basis, an unnecessary product test. That test would have added to the product cost without having any positive impact on product

safety or effectiveness. By seeking a clear understanding of the actual testing requirements, rather than blindly following the industry standard and normal testing guidelines designed for a different technology, the organization demonstrated equivalent
quality assurance and control without added expense or unnecessary and inappropriate additional testing.

The organization invested relatively little money in outside assistance to
develop a persuasive and well-supported case; it also discussed that case with the
FDA in a scheduled conference and presented the evidence (effectively and successfully) in the 510(k) application for the medical devices (plastic condoms).

ESTIMATED SAVINGS

Direct: $2,128,000

Indirect: no indirect

NOTES

The FDA's generally willingness to schedule briefings and meetings with client
organizations to discuss specific issues is a long-standing policy in the medical
device arena, much more recently extended to pharmaceutical and biologics regual-
tion. See *Guidebook to Drug Regulatory Submissions* (Weinberg: Wiley, 2009) for
detailed guidance regarding the requesting and scheduling of FDA conferences.

Regulation generally has an anti-innovative impact, since many organizations
are afraid to try a new approach that might either add unwelcomed regulatory scrutiny or overestimate the cost of compliance when evaluating the expenses of a
new technology. This hesitation to develop new technologies and approaches has a
negative impact on the idnustry and on the long-term public health. The industry
and the agency need to guard against this tendency. One executive recently reported,
for example, that his company had decided not to automate their laboratory since
the existing facility was compliant and the cost of validating a new LIMS was excessive. The result was greater costs in labor and maintenance, less reliable results, and
fewer available laboratory controls. It often seems that fear of the FDA, generally
unwarranted, is the major barrier in the pharmaceutical, device, and biologics
industries.

Case Code: B1ES

Case: Biologics Electronic Submission

Author: Rockburne

Industry: [ ] Pharma   [X] Biologics   [ ] Medical Device

Strategy: [ ] Requirements   [ ] Audits   [ ] Quality by Design

[ ] Outsource   [X] Electronic Submissions   [ ] EMEA Overlap

BACKGROUND

This major international pharmaceutical company headquartered in Illinois is a process of human plasma. The products include antibody and coagulation factors. The company has an excellent reputation, with the regulation authorities within the countries in which it is doing business. Fundamentally, the markets for the company's plasma product are within the United States and the European Community. The company has 39 employees primarily based in the United States, with an office in London to service the EC.

The Food and Drug Administration (FDA) is the Federal agency responsible for the blood industry by licensing products and issuing as well as enforcing safety rules. The Center for Biologics Evaluation and Research (CBER) is the FDA component responsible for regulating products used for the prevention, treatment, or cure of diseases and injuries including blood products.

The applicant must prepare a Biologic License Application (BLA), which is a document submitted to the FDA to request approval to market a biologic. The BLA is equivalent to an NDA for a biologic (biologic = a therapeutic DNA plasmid product, therapeutic synthetic peptide product of 40 or fewer amino acids, monoclonal antibody product for in vivo use, or therapeutic recombinant DNA-derived product).

The EMEA operates under the European legislative body requiring different regulatory procedures and has established the concept of a Plasma Master File (PMF). The PMF is a compilation of all the required scientific data on the quality and safety of human plasma relevant to the medicines, medical devices, and investigational products that use human plasma in their manufacture. The data cover all aspects of the use of plasma, from collection to plasma pool.

STRATEGIC ACTION

Upon reviewing the criteria that the company must meet if they are to move forward, it was decided by the company's Project Manager (Bob) to submit a BLA to the FDA as well as comply with the pertinent directive for the EMEA: to recommend to the Vice President of Regulatory Affairs (Tom) that it would be cost efficient to make concurrent/overlapping submissions to the FDA and EMEA.

Bob noted the following general strategic considerations:

- Concurrent submissions allow the use of one in-house approval process to bolster and support the second application.

- Concurrent applications significantly reduce the review time (overlapping the FDA and EMEA review periods), speeding the time to market and reducing costs.

- Concurrent applications ease the compliance management process, making Bob's job less complicated.

- Concurrent applications require complex electronic formatting to manipulate application sections into appropriate order and location for each application.

Furthermore, Bob made the decision to submit the required documentation to the respective regulatory bodies electronically. By so doing, his team could use the common data required by both the FDA and the EMEA. He would also make use of personnel in the company's London office to liaise with the EMEA.

Pertinent data common to both submissions would include detailed reports of product purity, safety, efficacy, control, history, and proper labeling. It would then become a straightforward exercise of reorganizing these reports to meet the FDA submission guidelines (BLA).

In a similar manner, the Company's e-submission to the EMEA would follow the guidelines established to make application to the Plasma Master File so that after successful review of the documentation the EMEA would issue a PMF Certificate, thereby allowing the company to market its product throughout the EC.

By following the concurrent plan, Bob calculated a reduction of time from the first submission (EMEA) through review and acceptance to the FDA submission of review and acceptance as follows:

−3.25 years to a total of 1.75 years (savings of 18 months: −300 business days) at patent/market gain of estimated $250,000 per day (300 days) = $75 million in indirect savings

EFFECT

Bob submitted his analysis of the simultaneous submission plan to Tom, the Vice President of Regulatory Affairs for the company. The implementation of the simultaneous submission strategy is based upon the development of a database of application sections that can be rearranged and modified to meet the unique requirements of the FDA and EMEA. Once this database is defined and established, future simultaneous applications are significantly simplified. For example, the BLA is submitted by any legal person or entity who is engaged in manufacture or an applicant for a license who takes responsibility for compliance with product and establishment standards. Form 356h specifies the requirements for a BLA. This includes:

- Applicant information
- Product/manufacturing information
- Preclinical studies
- Clinical studies
- Labeling

The review period for an FDA or EMEA application is approximately six months but could be in excess of a year, depending on the review of the data submitted to the respective agencies. Even with a longer one-time preparatory time (as opposed to separate preparations for the two agency applications), the adoption of a simultaneous strategy is likely to reduce the review by the nonoverlapping six months.

PROBLEMS/CHALLENGES

However, this organization faces a number of challenges, not the least of which is the compete unfamiliarity with the simultaneous submissions approach. In other words the learning curve was a bit more prolonged. Probably the most important challenge was dealing with the EMEA and FDA definitions of the requirements of the FDA relative to the BLA and the EMEA requirements relative to establishing a Plasma Master File. Second, the initial establishment of the sectional database required some time and investment that should be recovered as the simultaneous system is perfected. Finally the e-submission process per se was slightly different for both agencies. However, both agencies had excellent e-guiding systems that were a great assistance to the applicant.

None of the above problems proved to be insurmountable but would affect the economics of the method of approach. Given that the company does business in both the United States and the EC, this in-house expertise would prove to be invaluable.

COST CONTAINMENT

Utilizing the simultaneous submissions strategy (FDA and EMEA), the company was able to both reduce the preparatory costs the applications to the two regulatory agencies, but more importantly was able to significantly reduce the total review time of the two applications, resulting in real potential savings through control of patent period and a competitive speed to market. Although not a historical part of this particular case, further cost containment could potentially have been realized through simultaneous submissions to regulatory agencies in Canada, Brazil, Israel, Australia, and Switzerland (Japanese formatting and regulations are sufficiently distinct as to make this approach highly problematic).

As with any new strategy, the organization found some difficulties with initial implementation that they expected and that would be eliminated with greater experience with the simultaneous method of approach.

ESTIMATED SAVINGS

Direct: $50,000
Indirect: $75 million

NOTES

The development of this in-house capability presents several cost advantages for the company. First the ability to e-submit to a number of different regulatory agencies biologic products will give the company a significant cost advantge since they are principly using the format based on the International Conference on Harmonization

(ICH) Common Technical Document (CTD). The document is basically used outside of the United States.

Second, the time-related indirect savings result more from the competitive advantage of speed to market than from increased longevity of patent protection. Third, the use of a new simultaneous submission strategy requires a learning curve on the part of the company. It also encourages the company to form an in-house consulting arm to take advantage of a newly enhanced experience in strategy and expertise in the registration of biologic products with regulatory agencies.

The "bottom line" is that the company found significant savings in the simultaneous submission to both FDA and EMEA of registration of plasma product and in addition will open up new markets in other areas of the world.

CHAPTER 11

COST-CONTAINMENT ANALYSIS

11.1 INTRODUCTION

The ultimate test of any strategy is its effectiveness. No matter how elegant or well-packaged a strategy may be, it is worthless unless it helps to achieve the fundamental goals for which it was intended. The six strategies described here—the development of clear, unambiguous definitions of actual regulatory requires; the use of outside auditors to preempt and anticipate FDA visits; the implementation of an automated quality system using Quality by Design (QbD); the outsourcing of short-term or highly expert staff; the use of electronic rather than paper manual submissions; and the simultaneous submissions of approval documents to both the FDA and EMEA—are all intended to help contain the costs associated with regulation.

While these regulatory costs may not represent the majority expense in the development and production of pharmaceutical, biologic, and medical device products, they do represent the area most ready for reform. While quality is of top priority, it is a finite achievement goal. Inspecting a pacemaker for integrity of power source is an appropriate and prudent control; checking the same power source multiple times adds unnecessary expense without improving that quality. Since the role of regulation is the development of standards for and enforcement of standards related to self-implementation of appropriate quality levels, excessive or excessively expense regulation adds cost without value. In a finite economic world in which higher expenses, inevitably passed to consumers as higher product prices, is an impediment to public access to those products, unnecessarily excessive regulation reduces the availability of therapeutics, cures, and treatments in the most economically vulnerable tail of the population curve.

It is, of course, not necessary to rank order these cost-containment strategies. Some will be appropriate for some organizations and inappropriate for companies. Some strategies may work well in one period of time, but may be of lesser value under other circumstances. And some strategies may already be in place, but may be enhanced or increased to the benefit of the organization. Most importantly, these six strategies are not mutually exclusive. An organization could decide to outsource the development of simultaneous electronic submissions to EMEA and FDA, or it could combine a QbD strategy with the development of clear and unambiguous regulatory requirements.

But in order to justify any of these strategies, alone or in combination, to an upper management evaluation or an implementation team set of expectations, it is necessary to evaluate their relative effectiveness. How will each of the strategies contribute to cost containment? What expectations are appropriate?

11.2 THE STRATEGIES

The six cost-containment strategies—requirement definition, auditing, QbD, outsourcing, electronic submissions, and simultaneous EMEA submission—can be effectively evaluating according to five criteria:

Likelihood of Success in Containing Regulatory Costs: Is this strategy likely to be effective in a given organization (pharmaceutical, biologics, medical device)? Is it worth pursuing in Your organization?

Probable Direct Cost Savings: Based upon the author's field experience, what is the likely range of savings to be realized?

Probable Indirect Cost Savings: Based upon the author's field experience, what is the likely range of savings to be realized?

Area of Indirect Cost Savings: Are indirect savings a result of reducing time to approval and eventual market, to improved regulatory reputation, to improved efficiency in staff, or to other factors?

Probable FDA Conformance Satisfaction Level: With the implementation of the specific strategy, what is the likely FDA response?

Using these criteria, it is possible to examine each of the strategies in turn.

11.2.1 Requirements

The first strategy for containing regulatory costs involves developing documenting clear definitions for actual regulatory requirements, avoiding the exaggeration and inflation effects that so commonly increase the regulatory burden. By determining the appropriate quality level for a given situation—in effect, taking corporate responsibility for self-regulation—and providing both clear definitions and evidence of compliance, an organization can trim inappropriate requirements to a cost effective and manageable level.

The cost containment of such a strategy is clear. By replacing general and hence vague requirements with justifiable and specific standards, an organization can avoid the "overkill" phenomenon that drives up regulatory costs without improving human health and safety. While an organization may want to go a bit "beyond the line" for political or insurance reasons, knowing where that line actually is and by clearly defining its limits compliance can be achieved without exaggerated expense. Those expenses saved are direct and (depending on the organization) can be significant. While the evidence is not complete, there seems to be a correlation between the age and size of the organization and the costs that can be contained:

Apparently the longer an organization is in operation and the more diverse its activities, the more likely that the original requirements will drift and expand, leaving room of effective trimming. Even in new and focused organizations, though, the tendency to "build a wall around" perceived requirements leads to unnecessary and unintended (by regulatory authorities) extra effort and expense. Without the establishment of clear, situation-specific, and justified interpretations of general regulatory principles, additional unnecessary costs are likely to accumulate rapidly.

While variances are wide, experience with implementation of the "requirements" strategy suggest that by (a) developing specific and tightly defined internal standards that meet the spirit and letter of published regulatory requirements, (b) documenting those standards and the rationale supporting them, and (c) documenting compliance with those established standards, the average organization can reduce the required regulatory and quality assurance personnel in the range of two full-time persons—including overhead, a savings expectation of approximately $220,000 per year. In addition, the company should be able to further save the equivalent on one person by reducing the amount of unnecessary operating control activity, an additional $100,000 savings. Discounting the difficult to estimate but likely significant indirect savings accruing from more efficient operations, the "requirements strategy should produce an estimated $320,000 per year in cost containment.

Likelihood of Success in Containing Regulatory Costs: High. Experience suggests that most organizations aim for a compliance level well in excess of actual requirements.

Probable Direct Cost Savings: $100,000–$320,000 per annum.

Probable Indirect Cost Savings: Low.

Area of Indirect Cost Savings: Increased staff focus on actual requirements.

Probable FDA Conformance Satisfaction Level: High.

11.2.2 Auditing

Auditing requires an investment to eventually control costs. An extra step is added, falling between the documentation of compliance and the investigation of that documentation by the Food and Drug Administration: An independent auditor (in-house or external) conducts a review of the documentation and the situation it describes. That audit may then generate corrective actions, again reviewed by the auditor. Eventually, the auditor issues a report summarizing the compliance situation. That report in turn becomes the primary review document in a future FDA visit.

Because the organization has had an opportunity to take corrective action outside the regulatory spotlight, and because the result with regard to corporate reputation—the FDA correctly understanding that the company has assumed primary regulatory responsibility and is appropriately exercising that responsibility—is highly positive, the organization is likely to find itself with fewer fines or adverse findings. It is therefore less likely to suffer production delays resulting from regulatory actions in response to serious problems, and it is more likely to find a rapid response to submissions (particularly in approvals or amendments to production facilities and processes).

Adoption of an independent auditor strategy has proven to be very effective in organizations that have chosen this path, in all aspects of the FDA-regulated industries (pharmaceutical, biologics, and medical device). While not formally required by any FDA regulations, the auditor's report provides FDA visitation teams with a level of confidence that focuses the inspection of important high-level issues rather than minutiae of documentation or trivia. Because the inspection team has wide-ranging responsibilities, the members are unlikely to have real expertise in the system they are observing. They therefore tend, in the absence of an outside audit report, to fall back on areas of personal interest or on general issues of compliance to SOPs and clarity of documentation.

Likelihood of Success in Containing Regulatory Costs: Medium: little impact on direct costs (in fact, likely an increase in expenses) and difficult to document indirect savings.

Probable Direct Cost Savings: Zero or negative.

Probable Indirect Cost Savings: Increased regulatory confidence, corporate reputation, speed of approval of submissions.

Area of Indirect Cost Savings: Reputation for quality and for self-regulation.

Probable FDA Conformance Satisfaction Level: Very high.

11.2.3 Quality by Design

Quality by Design (QbD) is an evolving FDA-industry initiative that potentially results in the automation of some key quality control and assurance processes. Using the current QbD paradigm, an analysis is made of process to determine the potential degree and areas of quality risk; those key manufacturing (or other) variables are then assigned appropriate ranges of acceptable conformity using a design space analysis, based upon the risk analysis findings. Finally, each of the key variables is continuously monitored and, where possible, subject to cybernetic (self-correcting) control. The result is a self-regulation and monitoring process overseen by the automated system, presumably with periodic human review.

The cost containment flowing from QbD should be significant, flowing from two direct sources. First, an automated (or even semiautomated) quality control and assurance process should reduce required QA/QC headcount, producing salary and overhead benefits. Second, because the QbD process involves continuous cybernetics monitoring, it should significantly reduce the costs of discarded substandard product or product reprocessing. Indirect savings will result from increased regulatory reputation and from fewer recalls resulting from quarantine errors.

Unfortunately, the very early stage of QbD, largely experimental, precludes any meaningful quantification of these savings. Predictions of direct savings generally hover around $500,000 to $1 million (a very large range) but are notoriously problematic. And those savings are likely to be reduced by the investment costs incurred with a QbD system, yet to be determined.

Likelihood of Success in Containing Regulatory Costs: Very high, once the QbD system is perfected, agreed upon, and widely implemented.

Probable Direct Cost Savings: No accurate estimates.

Probable Indirect Cost Savings: No accurate estimates.

Area of Indirect Cost Savings: Reduced time to approval and eventual market; improved regulatory reputation; reduced likelihood of recalls due to quarantine errors.

Probable FDA Conformance Satisfaction Level: Very high.

11.3   OUTSOURCING

Outsourcing is the classic—and often misused—strategy for cost containment in all parts of an organization. As a regulatory approach, outsourcing can be effective in a situation in which (a) critical expertise and/or experience is missing, (b) that expertise/experience is needed for a short-term or finite project, (c) by using outsource experts the in-house team will gain the necessary skills to manage similar situations in the future, or (d)the involvement of a highly credible industry opinion leader will be of value for a specific issue or question. While outsourcing for other reasons such as reducing full-time headcount may meet other corporate goals, the use of long-term consultants is generally not an effective regulatory cost-containment strategy. Because of the confidential and legalistic nature of regulatory work, it is strongly recommended that long-term projects are managed by permanent employees.

Outsourcing can control costs through three mechanisms. First, because the consulting outsource employees are "1099" personnel (as defined by the Internal Revenue Service Code Section 1099), the hiring organization is not required to pay Federal taxes related to Medicare, Medicaid, workman's comprehensive insurance, unemployment insurance, and so forth—approximately 7% of the paid wages. This savings, plus savings in paid benefits (medical, retirement, vacation, etc.), may offset the consulting fees charged (generally higher than normal full-time employee wages).

Second, because effective and efficient outsourcing brings in needed expertise for a brief period, significant savings can be realized through the advantage of that expertise. Rather than "reinventing the wheel," an outsource SOP expert, submission expert, or clinical quality control expert may produce savings through efficiency and time-on-project reductions.

Third, the skills transfer that can result from including the outsource consultant on a mixed (employee and consultant) team can be a very efficient method of training full-time staff, resulting in greater effectiveness (and reduced need for outsourcing in the future). The result is likely to be cost containment through improved skill levels.

Together these three advantages can result in significant cost savings when outsourcing is utilized in an appropriate, short-term, expertise-enhancing manner.

Likelihood of Success In Containing Regulatory Costs: Very high (given the short-term use caveat).

Probable Direct Cost Savings: An average of 4% over the use of full-time employees.

Probable Indirect Cost Savings: High, a result of (a) improved efficiency through the gain of expertise and experience and (b) enhancement of in-house skills.

Area of Indirect Cost Savings: Reduced time to approval and eventual market, improved regulatory reputation.

Probable FDA Conformance Satisfaction Level: Very high.

11.4   ELECTRONIC SUBMISSIONS

The use of electronic submissions of key FDA documents has become increasingly commonplace, and the potential benefits of improved and more rapid regulatory review have increasingly been realized as FDA internal expertise has improved. To date, there are three strategic options for electronic submissions:

Electronic submissions in lieu of paper submission

Paper submission with electronic hyperlinks (hybrid)

Electronic submissions with paper backup submissions

In many FDA subgroups the first option is yet to be recommended; in some the suggested first choice is a paper submission with hyperlinks. Over time, however, the dream of fully electronic submissions will be achieved with resulting cost containment of shipping, preparation, indexing, copying, and other related expenses.

The cost containment achievable from transition from a paper or hybrid paper system to a purely electronic submission can be calculated with some precision. A recent consulting project involving preparation of IND and NDA submissions (pharmaceutical, neurological) included collection of both in-house and multiple (four) external bids for electronic, paper, and hybrid processes. The results averaged (with remarkably little variation):

Media	Ind	Nda
Electronic	$378,000	$1.24 million
Hybrid	$720,000	$1.58 million
Paper	$562,000	$1.54 million

Examining just the paper versus electronic submission differential suggests a direct savings of $184,000 (relatively minor submission, the IND) or $300,000 (major NDA submission).

Indirect savings accrue from increased speed of preparation of documents and of FDA review, as well as increase FDA appreciation of electronic submissions (currently largely limited to hyperlink features connecting text to references).

Likelihood of Success in Containing Regulatory Costs: Very high (assuming increasing FA familiarity with review of electronic submissions).

Probable Direct Cost Savings: $184,000 to $300,000.

Probable Indirect Cost Savings: High, increasing as in-house and FDA expertise grow.

Area of Indirect Cost Savings: Reduced time to approval and eventual market, improved regulatory reputation.

Probable FDA Conformance Satisfaction Level: High and increasing.

11.5   EMEA SUBMISSIONS

The EMEA Submissions strategy calls for developing a significant regulatory submissions document (IND, NDA, BLA, etc.) as a series of separate documents, each addressing a regulatory issue, and then assembling separate versions to meet the inclusion and organizational requirements of both the FDA and EMEA. This approach permits simultaneous rather than sequential submissions to the two agencies, resulting in a significant reduction in review time and a subsequent savings in speed to market and patent life.

The cost savings related to the EMEA Submissions strategy are mostly indirect. On a direct basis, there may be some slight savings in regulatory costs since both sets of documents are produced together, but that containment is lost in the cases where a rejection in the first application results in abandonment or major modification in the second. In effect the strategy saves expenses when successful, but increases costs when unsuccessful.

Because of the finite patent life and the lengthy FDA (and, to a lesser degree, EMEA) review time, simultaneous submission results in significant financial advantage in that reduced review time increases available market time under patent exclusivity. And more rapid time to market may result in other gains in market share and product choice. Generally the more rapid the move from clinical tests to public release, the greater the profitability of the drug, biologic, or medical device.

Likelihood of Success in Containing Regulatory Costs: Very high (assuming that the two applications are complete and appropriately structured.

Probable Direct Cost Savings: Minor, perhaps $50,000 in production costs of the two applications.

Probable Indirect Cost Savings: Very high, cutting years off the regulatory review process and hence expanding the period of patent protected market exclusivity.

Area of Indirect Cost Savings: Reduced time to approval and eventual market.

Probable FDA Conformance Satisfaction Level: High.

11.6   VARIANCES BY INDUSTRY

While the same cost-containment regulatory strategies work for the pharmaceutical, biologics, and medical device industries, there are some differences that make some strategies more success in certain settings.

The requirements strategy is successful for all three industries, but may prove to provide the greatest benefits to biologics organizations. Requirements may be less clearly defined in that sector, and hence the advantage of self-defining situation-specific requirements may be most noticeable. In the medical device industry, requirements have been generally clearly defined (in part because of their use of three classes of devices, with appropriately different requirements), and hence the strategic advantage will prove less dramatic.

The auditing strategy will be most accepted by (and hence most successful with) the medical device reviewers. As a result of the complexity of computerized medical devices the FDA has been generally accepting of audit reports they can review in lieu of more detailed agency investigations. To a lesser degree, the strategy will produce savings in the pharmaceutical sector, largely by producing fewer embarrassing adverse finding reports.

While QbD is still in its infancy, the greatest impact is likely to be in the pharmaceutical industry, where the production process is a significant focus of regulatory concerns. Biologics may also eventually adopt QbD strategies, particularly in defining and monitoring product purity. Application of the strategy to medical devices is more problematic (though see Case Q1D).

Outsourcing will prove successful cost containment for all three industries. Whenever human resources, expertise, and experience are lacking, the use of effective outsourcing can prove effective.

The switch to electronic submissions will save review time in all three industries, but the change will most significantly be felt in the pharmaceutical sector, where review procedures are most problematic. Lesser but still significant advantages will be seen in medical device and biologics industries.

The process of EMEA submission will prove highly effective in the medical device industry (where progress in harmonization has brought the two review processes into relatively close alignment) and in biologics where relatively similar procedures evolved simultaneously. Organizations applying the strategy to the pharmaceutical sector will find some advantages, but will likely see significant differences in the final submissions for the two agencies.

11.7 SUMMARY

While quantification is often problematic, particularly in assessing long-term benefits of the six identified regulatory cost-containment strategies, there is clear evidence that these approaches will prove useful in reducing the costs associated with compliance in the pharmaceutical, biologics, and medical device industries. The savings ultimately flow from a few near-universal business principles: Plan ahead, know your subject matter, minimize unnecessary headcount, and bring in expertise when needed.

In the heavily regulated industries of pharmaceutical, biologics, and medical device, maintaining product quality (and hence public safety) while minimizing costs (and hence public access to treatments and preventatives) is both good business and good public policy. These six strategies—establishment of clear situation-specific requirements; auditing to anticipate regulatory reviews; implementation of the quality automation offered by a QbD approach; the use of outsourcing to bring in temporary expertise and experience; the use of electronic rather than manual/paper submissions; and the simultaneous submission of documents to the FDA and EMEA—can together result in significant direct and indirect savings. The result is likely an improvement in quality coupled with a reduction in cost: successful achievement of the combined goal of greater public access to safer, higher-quality drugs, biologics, and medical devices.

CHAPTER 12

MANAGING REGULATION IN TIMES OF CHAOS

The United States Food and Drug Administration would never be described as nimble. It is closer in performance to a huge aircraft carrier, so massive as to require long advance preparation to change direction or significantly modify policy. Rarely, however, that lumbering giant does turn, and during the maneuver the result is likely to be chaos.

New regulations generally require about a two- to three-year change period, starting with the formation of a joint agency/industry committee, progressing through the announcement of a draft policy, proceeding through a comment and review period, and eventually ending with the release of a final guideline or regulation. The implementation and enforcement of that regulation may evolve over an additional two to five years, ultimately resulting in a new course for the FDA or one of its primary centers.

During this transition period of two to eight years, FDA field investigators, agency reviewers, industry experts, and supplementing consultants find themselves forced to operate on a combination of guess, rumor, and prayer. Everyone is aware that the old requirements are no longer in play, but the details of the new guidelines are unclear. The draft release is often misleading, generally reflecting much more radical change than the final result. Consultants may have incentives to exaggerate the forthcoming requirements and to promulgate the draft positions as if those pre- liminaries were final. Some agency people operate under the old original guidelines; others try to anticipate the forthcoming changes. And companies planning long-term strategies are left with confusion and the added expense of trying to support multiple possible outcomes.

These rare but significant periods of transitional chaos require special cost- containment strategies. This may affect all parts of the FDA—the Good Manufacturing Practices are due for revision shortly—or a specific segment of the industry. But for any organizations finding themselves in transition confusion, careful planning and the delicate balance of a ballerina are required.

Cost-Contained Regulatory Compliance: For the Pharmaceutical, Biologics, and Medical Device Industries, First Edition. Sandy Weinberg.
© 2011 John Wiley & Sons, Inc. Published 2011 by John Wiley & Sons, Inc.

12.1 THE 2009 MEDICAL DEVICE LETTER

In January of 2009 an informal collection of physicians and scientists in the US Food and Drug Administration's Center for Devices and Radiological Health (FDA–CDRH sent a letter to the Obama transition team. Bypassing multiple layers in the chain of command, "airing dirty laundry in public," and evoking the long taboo "corruption" word, these CDRH employees sent a lengthy letter to John Podesta, head of the Obama transition team, charging that the FDA was putting the nation's health at risk through inadequate policies and procedures.

The key paragraph stated:

> The purpose of this letter is to inform you that the scientific review process for medical devices at FDA has been corrupted and distorted by current FDA managers, thereby placing the American people at risk. ... This letter provides an inside view of the severely broken science, regulation and administration at the Center for Devices and Radiological Health (CDRH) that recently forced FDA physicians and scientists to seek direct intervention from the US Congress.

The specifications focused on two major themes: The first theme was that there was an antiquated policy of waiving clinical testing for devices that related to "predicates," even if those predicates had never been adequately tested. The end result was the revelation that many medical devices in widespread use in the United States had been approved without ever being subject to efficacy clinical testing, and that some of those devices had even bypassed safety clinical testing. The second theme was that top CDRH managers were "stacking" expert review panels, allowing disqualification of scientists for arbitrary reasons and ordering "physicians and scientists to ignore FDA Guidance Documents."

In response to the procedural question, indicting top FDA management for perceived undue influence, the Obama administration used the governmental transition to permit top FDA and CDRH personnel to resign or retire. The predicate policy issue is more complex, and is the subject of an ongoing revision of FDA guidelines for approving medical devices. And that policy revision is creating chaos within the medical device industry.

The letter itself is interesting in both the breadth and depth of its indictment, leading in turn to a period of chaos as procedures are subject to an extraordinary review (Figure 12.1).

All medical device submission and review policies are under review, with new interpretations expected over the next two to five years. In the first year after the letter that prompted reexamination of procedures, the FDA has announced a significant tightening of reviews of radiological devices and has formed task forces to examine (a) the use of predicate devices, (b) the 510(k) and Pre-Market Approval process, (c) the 510(d) exemptions, and (d) the formation of device review panels. As a result, medical device companies are torn between conflicting advice, fluid requirements, and uncertain strategies.

While the current chaos is focused on the medical device approval process, the same kinds of confusion can affect pharmaceutical companies, biologics organizations, and/or the industry as a whole. In 2001 the FDA released a significant

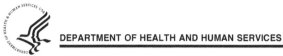

DEPARTMENT OF HEALTH AND HUMAN SERVICES

Food and Drug Administration
Center for Devices and Radiological Health
9200 Corporate Boulevard
Rockville, MD 20850

January 7, 2009

John D. Podesta
Presidential Transition Team
Washington, DC 20270

Dear Mr. Podesta:

We, physicians and scientists of the U.S. Food and Drug Administration (FDA), fully support the agenda of President Obama to "challenge the status quo in Washington and to bring about the knid of change America needs."[1] America urgently needs change at FDA because FDA is fundamentally broken, failing to fulfill its mission, and because re-establishing a proper and effectively functioning FDA is vital to the physical and economic health of the nation. As stated in the November 2007 FDA Science Board Report[2] entitled *FDA Science and Mission at Risk*: "A strong FDA is crucial for the health of our country. The benefits of a robust, progressive Agency are enormous; the risks of a debilitated, under-performing organization are incalculable. The FDA constitutes a critical component of our nation's healthcare delivery and public health system. The FDA, as much as any public or private sector institution in our country, touches the lives, health and well-being of all Americans. ... The FDA is also central to the economic health of the nation, regulating approximately $1 trillion in consumer products or 25 cents of every consumer dollar expended in this country annually. ... The importance of the FDA in the nation's security is similarly profound. ... Thus, the nation is at risk if FDA science is at risk."

The purpose of this letter is to inform you that the scientific review process for medical devices at FDA has been corrupted and distorted by current FDA managers, thereby placing the American people at risk. Through this letter and your action, we hope that future FDA employees will not experience the same frustration and anxiety that we have experienced for more than a year at the hands of FDA managers because we are committed to public integrity and were willing to speak out. Currently, there is an atmosphere at FDA in which the honest employee fears the dishonest employee, and not the other way around. Disturbingly, the atmosphere does not yet exist at FDA where honest employees committed to integrity and the FDA mission can act without fear of reprisal. This letter provides an inside view of the severely broken science, regulation and administration at the Center for Devices and Radiological Health (CDRH) that recently forced FDA physicians and scientists to seek direct intervention from the U.S. Congress.[3] This letter also provides elements of reform that are necessary to begin real change at FDA from the "bottom up."

Since May 2008,[4] the FDA Commissioner has been provided with irrefutable evidence that managers at CDRH have placed the nation at risk by corrupting and distorting the scientific evaluation of medical devices, and by interfering with our responsibility to ensure the safety and effectiveness of medical devices before they are used on the American public. Before a medical device can be cleared or approved by FDA, the law requires[5] that safety and effectiveness is determined based on "valid scientific evidence ... from which it can fairly and responsibly be concluded by qualified experts that there is reasonable assurance of the safety and effectiveness of the device." Managers at CDRH have ignored the law

Figure 12.1

and ordered physicians and scientists to assess medical devices employing unsound evaluation methods, and to accept non-scientific, nor clinically validated, safety and effectiveness evidence and conclusions, as the basis of device clearance and approval. Managers with incompatible, discordant, and irrelevant scientific and clinical expertise in devices for which they have the full authority to make final regulatory decisions, have ignored serious safety and effectiveness concerns of FDA experts. Managers have ordered, intimidated, and coerced FDA experts to modify scientific evaluations, conclusions and recommendations in violation of the laws, rules and regulations and to accept clinical and technical data that is not scientifically valid nor obtained in accordance with legal requirements, such as obtaining proper informed consent from human subjects. These same managers have knowingly tried to avoid transparency and accountability by failing to properly document the basis of their non-scientific decisions in administrative records. As examples of wrongdoing, the Director of the Office of Device Evaluation (ODE) has gone so far as to:

- Order physicians and scientists to ignore FDA Guidance documents;
- Knowingly allow her subordinates to issue written threats of disciplinary action if physicians and scientists failed to change their scientific opinions and recommendations to conform to those of management;
- Issue illegal internal documents that do not conform to the requirements of Good Guidance Practices,[6] are not publicly available, and, if followed, would circumvent science and legal regulatory requirements;
- Fail to properly document significant decisions in the administrative files;[7]
- Make, and allow, false statements in FDA documents;
- Allow manufacturers to market devices that have never been approved by FDA;
- Remove Black Box warnings recommended by FDA experts;
- Bypass FDA experts and fail to properly label devices; and
- Exclude FDA experts from participating in Panel Meetings[8] because manufactures "expressed concerns that [FDA experts] are biased."

For seven months, Dr. von Eschenbach and his Assistant Commissioner for Accountability and Integrity (Mr. Bill McConagha) have conducted a sham investigation resulting in absolutely nothing: no one was held accountable, no appropriate or effective actions have been taken, and the same managers who engaged in the wrongdoing remain in place and have been rewarded and promoted. Dr. von Eschenbach and Mr. McConagha failed to take appropriate or effective actions while the physicians and scientists who had the courage and patriotism to speak out, and who refused to comply with FDA management wrongdoing, have suffered severe and ongoing retaliation.[9] The failure of Dr. von Eschenbach and Mr. McConagha to take appropriate or effective actions has made them complicit in the wrongdoing,[10] has harmed the reputaions and lives of individual employees, and has unnecessarily placed the American public at risk.

In October 2008, the U.S. Congress was provided with the same evidence of wrongdoing that was given to the Commissioner. After Congress examined the evidence, the U.S. House of Representatives Committee on Energy and Commerce sent a letter to the FDA Commissioner dated November 17, 2008,[11] stating that they had "received compelling evidence of serious wrongdoing ... and well-documented allegations ... from a large group of scientists and physicians ... who report misconduct within CDRH that represents an unwarranted risk to public health and a silent danger that may only be recognized after many years ... and that physicians and scientists within CDRH who objected [to the misconduct] ... have been subject to reprisals."

Figure 12.1   (Continued)

Unfortunately, the preceding facts are only the latest examples of shocking managerial corruption, wrongdoing and retaliation at CDRH. Back in February 2002, a biomedical engineer at CDRH reported serious managerial misconduct to the current Director of ODE and ultimately filed an EEOC lawsuit in September 2004. After six long stressful years of hardship and litigation, a Judge issued a forty-two page *Decision and Findings of Fact*[12] concluding that: "the Agency promoted a hostile working environment ... permeated with derogatory comments and adverse employment actions" ... the Agency "failed to exercise any reasonable care to prevent and correct promptly the harassing behavior" ... the actions toward the engineer were "unconscionable" and "occurred openly within the FDA, unchecked, for over four years" ... that "FDA managers were aware and failed to take appropriate or effective corrective actions; but rather, demonstrated a systemic disregard for federal regulations as well as the FDA's own policies." The Judge further concluded: "supervisors [including the current Director of ODE] knew or should have known of the hostile work environment, but neither the supervisors nor the Agency did anything to correct the situation or prevent further discrimination" ... and "failed to exercise any reasonable care to prevent or correct the hostility of [managers] towards the Complainant." Shockingly, the current Director of ODE herself testified in court that she was aware of the "hostile work environment" but "did not want to get involved," thereby corroborating her complicity in the corruption and retaliation against this employee. These independent facts confirm the longstanding pandemic corruption that cries out for new leadership at FDA from the bottom up.

We are confident that new leadership from the bottom up will be a top priority of Mr. Daschle as the new Secretary of the Department of Health and Human Services (HHS). As Mr. Daschle has recognized,[13] the integrity of the FDA scientific review and decision-making process, where scientific experts make evaluations and recommendations, must be evidence-based and independent, insulated from improper influences. As a matter of fact, Mr. Daschle points to the 1998 FDA approval of mammography computer-aided detection (CAD) devices[14] as an example of a breakdown of the independent scientific review and decision-making process. These CAD devices were supposed to improve breast cancer detection on mammograms. As Mr. Daschle recognized, post-approval scientific publications revealed that actual clinical performance of these CAD devices did not improve breast cancer detection[15] and they were associated with increased patient recalls and unnecessary breast biopsies.[16] We note that the Agency knowingly approved these devices in 1998 even though there was no clinical evidence of improved cancer detection and, furthermore, the device was never tested in accordance with its intended use—one of the principal required elements for device approval.[17] Astoundingly, the approval was based on pseudo-science that consisted of unsubstantiated estimates of potential benefit using flawed testing. Use of these devices is a major public health issue as approximately 40 million mammograms are performed every year in the U.S.[18] Furthermore, as a failure of FDA post-approval monitoring, the FDA never carried out any post-marketing assessment or re-evaluation of the clinical performance of these devices, ignoring accumulating clinical evidence provided by independent research publications revealing that these devices were ineffective and potentially harmful when used in clinical practice.

FDA managers continue to fail to apply even the most fundamental scientific and legal requirements for the approval of these, and so many other, devices. These failures constitute a clear and silent danger to the American public. Since 2006, FDA physicians and scientists have recommended five times not to approve mammography CAD devices without valid scientific and clinical evidence of safety and effectiveness. Manufacturers of these devices have repeatedly failed to provide valid scientific and clinical evidence

Figure 12.1 *(Continued)*

demonstrating safety and effectiveness of these devices in accordance with the intended use as required by the law. These matters were the subject of a Radiological Devices Panel meeting in March 2008[19] at which independent outside experts ratified all of the scientific, clinical, and regulatory points of the FDA experts required for proper assessment of the safety and effectiveness of these devices. Despite this, in April of 2008, the Director of ODE ignored the recommendations of all of the experts and approved these devices without any scientific, clinical or legal justification. Although unknown to Mr. Daschle and the American public, the Director of ODE and her subordinates committed the most outrageous misconduct by ordering, coercing, and intimidating FDA physicians and scientists to recommend approval, and then retaliating when the physicians and scientists refused to go along. This, and similar management actions with other devices, compelled us to write the FDA Commissioner in May 2008 and, because he utterly failed to take appropriate or effective actions, we later informed the U.S. Congress in October 2008.

We, physicians and scientists at FDA, seek your immediate attention for change and reform at FDA. To bring real change and reform to FDA, it is absolutely necessary that Congress pass, and the President[20] sign, new legislation providing the strongest possible protections for all government employees,[21] especially physicians and scientists, who speak out about wrongdoing and corruption that interferes with their mission and responsibility to the American public. We desperately need honesty without fear of retaliation for our evaluations and recommendations on medical devices, as well as accountability and transparency, to become the law and thus the foundation of the FDA mission and workplace. We totally agree with the following statement of President Obama:[22] "Often the best source of information about waste, fraud, and abuse in government is an existing government employee committed to public integrity and willing to speak out. Such acts of courage and patriotism, which can sometimes save lives and often save taxpayer dollars, should be encouraged rather than stifled. We need to empower federal employees as watchdogs of wrongdoing and partners in performance. Barack Obama will strengthen whistleblower laws to protect federal workers who expose waste, fraud, and abuse of authority in government. Obama will ensure that ... whistleblowers have full access to courts and due process."

As President Obama has emphasized, he intends to govern the nation and to bring about change from the bottom up. We believe that, as applied to FDA, this means a complete restructuring of the evaluation and approval process such that it is driven by science and carried out by clinical and scientific experts in their corresponding areas of expertise who are charged with review of regulatory submissions in accordance with the laws, rules and regulations. It is necessary that FDA expert physicians and scientists approve final regulatory determinations of safety and effectiveness, rather that multiple layers of managers who are not qualified experts and who often ignore scientific evidence and the law. President Obama has also emphasized the need for complete transparency in government. His Transparency Policy[23] should be mandatory for all FDA regulatory decisions and associated documentation. The long-standing FDA practice of secret meetings and secret communications between FDA managers and regulated industry must be strictly prohibited. Complete transparency in the regulatory decision-making process would serve as a deterrent to wrongdoing and an incentive for excellence.

FDA also requires major renovation of the organizational structure of the various Centers and Offices to restore internal checks and balances that proactively prevent corruption and manipulation of facts, science, and data. At present, FDA is plagued by a heavy-layered top-down organizational structure that concentrates far too much power in isolated Offices

Figure 12.1   (Continued)

run by entrenched managers where cronyism is paramount. We recommend that the Office of Device Evaluation be dismantled and split into multiple Offices, each headed by a physician or scientist with strong leadership credentials and extensive clinical and technical expertise in the specific devices they regulate. These leadership positions should be rotated on a regular basis. Furthermore, the current system of employee performance evaluation must be eliminated because it is used as an instrument of extortion by management and to terrorize employees who would otherwise serve as "watchdogs of wrongdoing and partners in performance."[24] The performance of FDA physicians and scientists must be based on an independent peer review process where extramural experts review the quality of the scientific content of their regulatory work.

We strongly support the sentiments expressed in a recent letter from Congressman Bart Stupak[25] urging complete change in FDA's current leadership. At CDRH, such change can be implemented immediately by removing and punishing all managers who have participated in, fostered or tolerated the well-documented corruption and wrongdoing. All improper management actions, including improper adverse personnel actions, and clearance/approval of medical devices that were not made in accordance with the laws, rules and regulations, must be reversed. Such swift and decisive action of transparency and accountability will send a strong message FDA-wide that wrongdoing will no longer be tolerated. In order to have a truly fresh start, we recommend that the new Commissioner request resignations from management positions by all current managers within CDRH, and use a competitive merit-based process to re-fill all management positions.

The FDA mission is not limited to premarket evaluation of safety and effectiveness. FDA is also responsible for the total product life cycle including actual clinical performance.[26] FDA must not engage in a fire-fighting regulatory posture after medical products are introduced into clinical practice and used on patients.[27] FDA must pursue a culture of proactive regulatory science and remain vigilant in monitoring clinical performance of devices. For FDA to fully accomplish its post-marketing responsibilities there must be complete coordination between FDA and all HHS health-related agencies and institutes.[28] This will provide FDA with the necessary critical scientific capability and capacity[29] to achieve its post-marketing oversight. In turn, FDA will be able to provide the American public and all health care decision makers with objective and scientifically rigorous assessments that synthesize available evidence on diagnosis, treatment and prevention of disease. Ultimately, this will result in a lower health care burden on our society.

In a time of transition, with the country facing an economic crisis with potential devastating consequences to the American people, we strongly believe that change and reform at FDA must be a top priority because FDA is central to the physical and economic health of the nation and because it can play a central role in reducing the future healthcare burden and avoiding public health catastrophes.[30] We sincerely hope that, together, we can establish a culture of science, honesty, transparency and integrity at FDA to serve as the genesis of reform for the entire American health care system.

Sincerely,

Figure 12.1   (Continued)

new guideline that presumably applied to all computer systems used in clinical support by any FDA-regulated organization. That new regulation—21 CFR Part 11—had been 20 years in development. Within months of its release, the FDA rescinded the regulation—an unprecedented action—and, half a year later, released a final revised version (with the addition of the risk concept included). In this example the intervening chaos affected aspects of the pharmaceutical, biologics, and device industries.

While the cost-containment strategies described in previous chapters have general applicability to all FDA situations, periods of chaos require consideration of additional, "special case" strategies as supplements to the risk, QbD, auditor, and other strategies described. There are four of these secondary strategies appropriate for consideration: duck and cover; shock and awe; delay; and confer. All four may be used in different situations, and they may be used in combination with any of the major cost containment strategies. While these four secondary approaches may not totally mitigate the chaos of emerging new regulations and guidelines, they can help an organization to cope and to survive the transition.

12.2 DUCK AND COVER

In the 1950s and 1960s, American school children were drilled in a maneuver called "duck and cover" as a response to an expected imminent nuclear attack. The strategy required that students climb under their desks and cover their heads with their arms. Luckily the action was never actually required; it is hard to imagine how it would have helped if a bomb were to vaporize the school. The strategy is no more effective than the mythical ostrich buying its head in the sand.

"Duck and Cover" is one possible strategy for coping with the chaos of rapidly changing FDA regulations; and while not always the best approach, it may prove more effective that climbing under a desk. Translated into a business strategy, "duck and cover" simply suggests that the best response to a period of confusion is no response at all. During regulatory transitions, an organization may be best served by not developing or submitting for marketing approval any new products, relying instead on the fine-tuning (within prenegotiated labels and designs) of existing products.

Consider two circumstances. In the first example, a company has been successfully marketing an approved product and has developed an improved replacement or enhancement that falls outside the scope of the original approval. In normal conditions the submission of evidence of safety and effectiveness of the new product would be reviewed according to established standards and either approved or rejected with a request for additional data. In either case, the organization could continue to market the original product while awaiting approval of the replacement.

In transition periods, however, review committees find themselves operating without clear guidance or criteria. While it is possible that the groups response will be to loosen requirements and approve normally rejected applications, the conservative bias of the FDA (and, arguably, of government-led committees) is more likely to result in a more careful and deliberate review.

Experience suggests that such review committees, seeking clarification of emerging standards, often examine the review procedure from previous products, in effect re-reviewing the existing product in hope of finding guidance for the new review. The result could well be a rescinding of the approval of the product on the market, now reexamined under vague or poorly established standards. Instead of finding itself with an established product while awaiting approval of the replacement, a company may find itself having to defend or recall the preapproved product in the face of chaotic reinterpretation of requirements.

Alternately, in scenario two, an organization has developed or discovered a product for which it has no previous market position. In this case, the review committee is likely to be left without any template or guidance for its analysis. Again, one result is rapid approval, but conservative committees are more likely to respond with a safer process: a long list of objections and questions, each likely to lead to additional requests for data or clarification.

Of course, it may seem that such a situation, while not desirable, is no worse than making no submission; presumably the committee will eventually run out of stalling questions and will eventually approve the new product. But should the new regulations be approved in the interim, the committee is likely to continue its review under the old vague situation, and it will await responses and requested data even if the new requirements do not necessitate that information. Submitting during the period of chaos may result in a longer review process than awaiting the release of the new requirements and submitting months or years later. The scenario makes a strategy of "duck and cover" very tempting.

During the first Gulf War the United States and Coalition Military adopted a strategy termed "shock and awe." The concept was to attack with such overwhelming force as to cause a rapid collapse of opposition. In the chaos of a new FDA regulatory revision, a "shock and awe" strategy may prove equally effective.

The approach requires a careful analysis of all potential requirements that might conceivably emerge from the new requirements under development. Often the first draft of the new guidelines can provide the core for this analysis: It represents the committee's dreams of regulatory control before the realities imposed by feedback and comments force more practical compromise. Once the possible requirements have been identified, the organization provides relevant evidence for all remotely likely regulatory requests, clearly identifying the evidence that demonstrates control under the previous (due for replacement) requirements and the supporting documentation that demonstrates conformity to possible new requirements.

Presumably, the submissions review committee or visiting investigator will be so impressed and overwhelmed with the depth and extent of the evidence, provided that approval or acceptance will come rapidly. While competitors have their heads buried in a "duck and cover" mode, the "shock and awe" strategies can obtain approval even in a time of chaos.

There are two important disadvantages of this "shock and awe" approach, however. First, it is an expensive strategy, requiring the extensive time and effort necessary to gather supporting information and to implement controls that are likely to prove unnecessary under the final emerging regulation. The organization may impose standard operating procedures, quality reviews, and tests that are not required under the final guidelines.

In the late 1980s, for example, the FDA began a long and lengthy review of system validation and control procedures for data analysis computer hardware and software. The final requirements, which did not emerge for 12 years, ignored hardware controls and minimized software testing. But in that interim many companies adopted their own internal validation requirements calling for extensive testing of hardware, operating systems, and networks. They met—actually significantly exceeded—the final requirements, but invested significant effort and funds in control procedures that were never actually required. And because of the sloth-like nature of many mega corporations, some organizations are still operating under their own overly burdensome "shock and awe" standards long after the FDA began requiring and permitting much more nimble and reasonable checks.

Second, the same field investigators and submissions review committee members that receive the "shock and awe" overly extensive body of evidence and control are likely to be involved in the rewriting of regulations and guidelines. When these individuals observe the depth and extent that organizations are prepared to submit, they are more likely to reject draft comments suggesting that the first version of the new regulation is overly burdensome, and they are more likely to include otherwise unnecessary requirements in the final document. The fact that they have seen the "shock and awe" quantity of supporting data makes the collection of that data all the more practical. During a time of chaos, the organizations opting for "shock and awe" may actually be moving along their own approvals at the cost of years of unnecessary additional regulatory burdens.

12.3   THE ACCESS FACTOR

Before examining the remaining two chaos strategies, it is appropriate to revisit the issue of public access to treatments, therapies, cures, and preventatives. The US FDA, along with regulatory agencies around the world, has been established to perform a delicate juggling act. Regulators must balance two often contradictory goals: (1) assuring the safety and efficacy of drugs, biologics, and devices and (2) providing the public with ready access to those products. In the United States with a mixed private/public payer system of health care, access generally translates to cost. The more expensive a therapy is, the less likely an insurance carrier will be able to absorb the expense, and the less likely a private payer will be able to afford the cost.

Because of the finite duration of a patent and the need to recover research and development investments before patent expiration permits generic companies to drop the profit margins, any delay in that development process can be very expensive. Millions of dollars in recovered expenses can be lost per day of delay. Those losses are ultimately passed on to consumers, resulting in higher product costs and reduced access to treatments and therapies.

So in times of regulatory revision and chaos, as (less dramatically) in normal times, delays in clinical research, regulatory review, submission, and other steps in the process result in reduced revenue for further research and increased product costs, both producing a reduction of access. In chaotic times, then, the FDA's natural conservative default is likely to swing the pendulum toward safety rather than access, and delays in the regulatory process are likely to push that pendulum further away from lower costs and increased public access to new drugs, biologics, and medical devices.

12.4 DELAY

Perhaps the natural reaction to a period of major revision and rewrite of regulatory requirements is simply to delay submissions and regulatory processes until the chaos has been quieted and new definitions of requirements have emerged. Small companies, ready to market single products, may not have that luxury. Large organizations, however, could potentially elect to slow their pipelines and to emphasize marketing of already approved products (perhaps to expanded label applications or with minor modifications). During revisions of drug regulations, for example, the large pharmaceutical companies focus on expanding applications of existing products and on introducing fast-dissolving, slow-dissolving, and other variations on already approved drugs.

Because of capital requirements, pharmaceutical development and manufacturing companies tend to be large (and well-funded), devices organizations tend to be small and minimally capitalized, and biologics companies (which often have the US government as their major customer) tend to fall in between. In the current medical device chaotic situation, then, pressures to minimize delays are intense: When new drug Good Manufacturing Practices are introduced, large drug companies may well opt for a one- to two-year gap in new drug developments and submissions.

Ultimately, however, both the large and small organizations have to carefully analyze the costs of delay against the lost revenue as patent periods are effectively shortened.[1] In the short run a strategy of delaying new product reviews until guidelines are released and promulgated throughout the agency is a tempting alternative. If the chaotic period is extensive, however, the delay may prove too costly and the strategy loses attractiveness.

Consider, again, the medical device situation. The public letter calling for major reform was released in January of 2009, resulting in a major internal revision that would normally result in new guidelines sometime in 2010 or 2011. As this chapter is in draft, however, the FDA Center for Radiological Health and Devices has announced the decision to hold public meetings to consider the direction of those changes (organized in February of 2010), presumably delaying that revision process until 2012 or 2013. Medical devices companies are likely facing a three- to five-year period of chaos—generally a period too long to permit a strategy of delay.

Similarly, the system validation period of confusion, measured from first public announcements of FDA concern for data quality controls (1986) until the introduction of the revised, risk inclusive version of 21 CFR Part 11 (2002), encompassed 16 years, at least 10 of which were characterized by confused interim guidelines contradictory advice from industry consultants and the FDA, and general chaos. Of course, these examples represent the extreme cases, but are sufficiently frequent to suggest that a delaying strategy, while attractive on the surface, may have significant disadvantages in certain circumstances.

---

[1]Note that the US Freedom of Information Act coupled with the prior disclosure prohibitions on patents effectively forces companies to file patents prior to initial FDA filings (presumable the IND or IDE), so that the patent exclusivity period is generally already running, and will continue to run, during any delay in clinical research and submission.

If, however, the period of revision is limited to 6–12 months (probably the minimum timeframe for a new guideline), simply awaiting the new release may be a viable and successful approach. And, of course, if a drug, biological, or medical device exists, the design or development pipeline in the middle or latter third of the chaotic period may prove a cost-effective solution.

12.5 CLARIFICATION (PRECONFERENCES)

The fourth potential strategy for coping with FDA regulatory chaos involves "forcing" a directly applicable interpretation of function guidelines for a specific project. It is largely applicable to submissions situations (IND, IDE, NDA, ANDA, PMA, BLA), though a modification can serve to a lesser degree in the event of investigator visits.

The Center for Radiological Health and Devices (CRHD) has scheduled conferences in advance of study launch or submission of data ever since its founding; Drug and Biologics centers (CDER and CBER) have followed suit for the last 10 years. The purpose of these conferences is to discuss the intended clinical study plan, submission strategy, or related issues and to achieve agreement between the agency and the specific industry group prior launching a major effort. The meetings generally are preceded by the submission to the FDA of a briefing book identifying the plan and the issues to be discussed, and they are followed by a formal or informal memorandum of agreement outlining the FDA's positions on those issues.

While the results of the meeting are not formally binding of the FDA (in case circumstances change or new regulations emerge), the agency generally is careful to abide by its agreements, which in effect serve as situation specific guidelines. Based upon this approach, it is possible to use the preconference procedure to (a) obtain clarification of the specific requirements to which a submission will be held and (b) define for that situation the regulatory standards—prerevision, draft, final revision, or whatever—that will be used to evaluate the result. The regulatory meeting, then, can be used to cut through the chaos for a specific case and to obtain industry–agency agreement on the interpretations that will apply to specified circumstances.

There are, of course, some limitations. In order to avoid finding itself swamped with numerous preconferences and to avoid being placed in the situation in which the FDA is used as an industry consultant, the agency limits the number of conference in which it will participate. Generally, a major submission is permitted one opportunity to discuss key questions; a second meeting is generally refused.[2] If a preconference had taken place before a new regulation was introduced or if an existing guideline had been revised or rescinded, it may not be possible to schedule a

---

[2] Incidentally, if the FDA finds itself in agreement with the all of questions raised in the Briefing Book, it may refuse the initial meeting, in which case the briefing interpretations stand. For this reason it is highly recommended that the briefing questions take the form of "Does the agency agree?" rather than "What does the FDA think?"

second meeting to cope with the new chaotic circumstances. The one meeting is very likely all that will be granted regardless of changing conditions.

And while prestudy or presubmission conferences are common, previsit or pre-investigation meetings are not. When the FDA arrives on site—generally unannounced (in the United States)—it may be possible to begin the visit with a discussion focusing, at least in part, on the specific regulations or interpretations to be used as criteria in the investigation. The most successful strategy for assuring such a discussion is to include it as a procedure in a Standard Operating Procedure for Audits and Regulatory Visits, prominently posted in the site lobby and provided to the FDA representatives when they identify themselves. But while this discussion may avoid some unproductive arguments and focus the guidelines of the investigation, the fact that it takes place immediately before walk through and document reviews provides little or no time to modify file organizations and procedural definitions in response to the regulatory interpretations and versions. Should the visitation team inform the organization management that it is seeking to know whether the company conforms to the 2004 interpretation of 21 CFR Part 11, for example, a company using newly emerging guidelines is unlikely to have the opportunity to reorganize supporting evidence in support of those guidelines. Still, it is no doubt better to know the interpretation being used than to not know, and the pre-inspection conference can help in the process.

While a preconference will not eliminate all transition confusion and may not clear away all kinds of regulatory chaos, it is often a valuable tool for coping with periods of change. The conference does not establish precedent transferable to other situations, but can at least clarify requirements for a unique and important set of circumstances.

12.6 SUMMARY

In times of regulatory transition resulting from rescinding, revision, or review or replacement of major guidelines and requirements documentation, confusion over what regulations are in current force can result in chaos. Four successful strategies for coping with these unusual circumstances can be considered: The selection of best approach or combination of approaches is a diopathic decision dependent upon issues of timing, access, and other special characteristics. Success has been had, however, with strategies of "duck and cover," "shock and awe," delay, and the use of conference meetings to obtain situation-specific guidance. A combination of all four approaches should be considered in determining the best approach for dealing with periods of regulatory chaos.

CHAPTER 13

INTERNATIONAL REGULATION

13.1   INTRODUCTION

The United States Food and Drug Administration (US FDA) dominates the United States' domestic drug, device, and biologics regulation. The agency also has great global influence, since the US market is highly attractive to international companies, and the US FDA represents a barrier to their entry into that market. But other national and international regulatory agencies are also at work protecting the populations of their countries, and an effective cost-controlled regulatory strategy addresses the concerns of these agencies as well. Here, then, is a list of the 12 major and most active non-US regulatory bodies, with summaries of focus and philosophy and follow-up contact information.

Many pharmaceutical, medical device, and biologics companies operate globally, so an analysis of the regulatory agencies and philosophies outside the United States is appropriate. In order to help determine how to apply the cost-containment strategies described in this text without other national boundaries, a comparison of these other regulatory environments to the US FDA is provided.

13.2   AUSTRALIA

13.2.1   Description of the Therapeutics Goods Administration (TGA)

Drugs, devices, and biologics produced and/or sold in Australia are regulated by the Department of Health and Ageing, Therapeutic Goods Administration (TGA). The TGA is established with the responsibility of "safeguarding the public health and safety in Australia by regulating medicines, medical devices, blood and tissues." The agency operates a prior registration system (Australian Register of Therapeutic Goods, ARTG), safety monitoring programs, alerts and advisories, and similar programs parallel to the USFDA. Areas of responsibility are restricted to medicines (including over-the-counter), medical devices, and blood and tissues. The agency also has some responsibility for the control of advertising, cosmetics, IVDs, and

Cost-Contained Regulatory Compliance: For the Pharmaceutical, Biologics, and Medical Device Industries, First Edition. Sandy Weinberg.
© 2011 John Wiley & Sons, Inc. Published 2011 by John Wiley & Sons, Inc.

"complementary medicines" (orphan drugs). The TGA does not have responsibility for food products.

Philosophically, the TGA tends to view itself more as a partner to industry rather than the oversight and barrier attitude of the USFDA. The organization provides guidance to industry to assist in moving through the approval process, and it often cooperates on the design of clinical trials. TGA utilizes a risk management approach, focusing product review and regulation on areas of greatest threat the public health and safety.

Importing therapeutic drugs for commercial purposes is restricted to product approved as listed on the ARTG. Australia has, however, reached cooperative agreements with some other regulatory bodies, including the EMEA.

Electronic submissions of regulatory applications and data are encouraged. Some user fees are charged to supplement government funding.

Australia has adopted Good Manufacturing Practices that are closely parallel to the EMEA cGMPs and that roughly approximate the US FDA cGMPs plus 21 CFR Part 11.

13.2.2 Pharmaceutical–Medical Device–Biologics Business in Australia

Australia has a relatively modest but mature home-grown pharmaceutical industry, with a heavy research emphasis on veterinary diseases (regulated outside the TGA). Australian universities have strong research and development programs that often work in cooperation with EMEA partners.

Doing business in Australia is efficient and streamlined, free of corruption and effectively supported by government agencies. The TGA has proven an effective promoter as well as regulator of business development, offering a variety of training programs and regulatory assistance guidance. While the tax structure in Australia may seem complex to American companies, the general business environment is healthy with strong government cooperation.

13.2.3 Differences Between US FDA and TGA

Australian regulation differs from the US regulatory environment in three important ways. First, note that the TGA combines some of the functions of the Centers for Disease Control and Prevention (CDC) and the National Institutes of Health (NIH) with the FDA in one agency. The TGA reports on disease outbreaks, the effectiveness of vaccine campaigns, and adverse drug reactions, and it provides some research activities and funding (particularly for orphan drug development).

Second, TGA attitude is much less adversarial than that of the USFDA. The agency has health promotion responsibilities as well as regulatory restriction authority and is much more likely to partner with researchers from industry to help bring a new drug, device, or biologic to market.

Third, while the TGA and FD greatly overlap in responsibility, note that the TGA does not have food or veterinary authority (and has only limited control of cosmetics). This restriction may help the Australian agency focus its attention on human medicines and therapies.

13.2.4   Summary

TGA is a modern, effective health and safety regulatory agency built on the European model of industry cooperation and oversight. Regulations (particularly cGMPs) and general procedures roughly parallel USFDA approaches, and a joint agreement with EMEA is currently in effect. The agency is relatively scandal-free, well-regarded, and professional.

13.2.5   TGA Follow-Up Contact Information

- Email: info@tga.gov.au
- Phone:
  - 1800 020 653 (free call within Australia)
  - 02 6232 8444 (switchboard)
  - 02 6232 8610 (for publications enquiries)
- Fax: 02 6203 1605
- Post: TGA, PO Box 100, Woden ACT 2606, Australia

13.3   BRAZIL

13.3.1   Description of the Sanitary Surveillance Agency (ANVISA)

Anvisa is a relatively new regulatory agency, first established in 1999. It falls under the Ministry of Health, and it coordinates with the National Sanitary Surveillance System (SNVS), the National Program of Blood and Blood Products, and the National Program of Prevention and Control of Hospital Infections. Anvisa also has responsibility for monitoring drug and device prices, as well as for providing technical support in patent review by the National Institute of Industrial Property. Interestingly, Anvisa was one of the first pharma regulatory bodies to be given responsibility for the control of tobacco products. Responsibilities include drugs, devices, and biologics, along with food, cosmetics, the aforementioned tobacco, and health services.

Anvisa has suffered since its first organization from a shortage of professional talent. Too few research scientists and qualified evaluators are stretched too thin in an agency with very broad responsibilities. The result has been complaints of inefficiency, corruption, and ineffectiveness. Anvisa attempts to work with industry to promote new product development, but often lacks the human resources to offer much real assistance and is criticized for the ways in which it selects those products and organizations to assist.

Brazil has monitored and participated in international cooperative programs, including the World Trade Organization (WTO), CODEX, and Merosul, and is negotiating harmonization of regulations and internationalization of technical requirements. To date no joint agreements have been announced.

Brazil operates on a very limited set of Good Manufacturing Practices, relying very heavily on an organization's internal practices as the standard of operation. The procedure for submitting and reviewing a drug for approval is only a few pages in length and gives little detail:

Procedures Manual for Registration of New Medicines

Documents Required for Registration of a New Product. This is applicable to those products falling within the following categories:

1. A product resulting from:
   (a) An alteration in the concentration of active substance or of its pharmacokinetic properties.
   (b) An active substance not registered for the purpose for which it was intended.
   (c) Withdrawal of the active component of a product already registered.
   (d) Substitution of the active component of a product already registered.
2. A product resulting from new molecular entities.
3. A new salt, despite the corresponding molecular body having already been authorized.
4. Two or more active unregistered substances, combined in the same product.

List of Documents Required for Registration

Document 01: Application forms FP1 and FP2, completed, as appropriate, in original plus one copy.

Document 02: Receipt (original plus one copy) proving payment of fee based on the Government Tariff, duly authenticated and/or stamped.

Document 03: Copy of the published announcement confirming award of Company Operating License.

Document 04: Receipt proving registration of the product, together with its original printed inserts (directions for use, etc.), approved in the country of origin and in other countries if applicable.

Document 05: Report of Therapeutic Testing, drafted and submitted in accordance with the sequence required according to Resolution 01/88 of 5/1/89, of the National Health Council, paying particular attention to the product's bioavailability and toxicity.

Document 06: Technical Report on the product containing the following items:

1. General data:
   (a) Pharmaceutical form in which it is presented.
   (b) Formula, indicating the basic components per dose required or, if possible, per gram, m/liter or standard international unit of measure.
   (c) Directions on how to administer/use product.
   (d) Main features, purpose, or use to which product is to be put.
   (e) Complementary therapeutic indications.
   (f) Contraindications, side effects, adverse reactions.

    (**g**) Restrictions or precautions that need to be considered.

    (**h**) Expiry date.

    (**i**) Storage precautions.

    (**j**) Instruction for use, if appropriate.

2. Pharmacodynamics:

    (**a**) How it works.

    (**b**) Dosage (maximum and minimum doses).

    (**c**) Justification for recommended doses.

3. Production and Quality Control:

    (**a**) The complete formula of the preparation, with all its components specified by the technical names, equivalent names, and synonyms in accordance with Brazilian Common Terminology (DCB), with the amounts of each substance expressed in metric units of measurement or in standard units, also denoting the substances used as a vehicle or excipient.

    (**b**) The production process, with a concise description of the various procedures to be carried out.

    (**c**) Descriptive report referring to quality control, based upon the active components of the formula of the product, together with stability and physio-chemical tests on the raw material and the finished product.

    (**d**) The tolerance limits for the tests and dosages, in the absence of official norms.

    (**e**) The code or method used by the company for identification of the shipment groups or batches of the product.

    (**f**) Report containing the technical data indicating no physical or chemical incompatibility between the packaging to be used and the components of the formula of the product.

    (**g**) Storage and transport precautions to be taken.

4. Complementary data:

    (**a**) Mention the registration of the substance or the basic components of the formula in the pharmacopoeia, in official publications dealing with pharmaceutical standards and/or in journals of scientific repute.

    (**b**) Enclose the bibliography on the product and the relevant literature; in the event of the product being of foreign origin, enclose a full translation from the original language. DETEN/SVS can request such information to be supplied (in duplicate for retention in its records), which it judges necessary for assessing the scientific documentation.

    (**c**) If the product contains narcotic, hypnotic, or barbituric substances, provide evidence indicating that the special provisions covering such substances have been complied with.

    (**d**) Demonstrate the advantages of the proposed formula, with a justification from a clinical standpoint.

(e) Other details that are appropriate or necessary, including those that elucidate causes and effects, in order to enable the health authorities to come to a correct conclusion about the product.

Document 07: Examples of the labels, printed inserts, typed in duplicate.

Document 08: Copy of the Operating License of the Company and/or its Health Permit.

Document 09: Written evidence that the manufacturing plant is overseen by the properly qualified responsible Technical Officer.

Additional Documents Required

In addition to the aforementioned documents, and depending on the product to be registered, the following procedure must be followed, in this order:

Document A: Copy, photocopy, or transcript of the registered permit in the country of origin in the case of drugs, medicines, or pharmaceutical inputs of foreign origin.

Document B: A report containing the recommendations, contraindications, and warnings presented with the application for registration in the country of origin signed by the Technical Officer responsible for the product to be registered.

Document C

The Good Practices Manual Used by the Company

Observations

(a) All the documentation must be signed by the Legal Representative of the company in question

(b) Documentation referring to the technical aspects of the application must in addition be signed by the Technical Officer responsible.

(c) The documents that have already been the subject of the Health Permit authorization do not need to be submitted.

While no doubt Anvisa will develop increasing sophisticated (and, alas, more complex) requirements and procedures over time, the current shortage of in-house expertise and experience has restricted the effectiveness of the agency. The current focus seems to be on registration of generic drugs, with little attention paid to the more complex process of developing and reviewing new drugs, devices, and biologics.

Anvisa's Mission: "To protect and promote health, ensuring the hygiene and safety of products and services and taking part in developing access to it."

13.3.2 Pharmaceutical–Medical Device/Biologics Business in Brazil

The current business environment seems to be focusing on the manufacturing and production of drugs and biologics for export to the US market. Anvisa has, for all practical purposes, delegated the regulation of these manufacturing facilities to the

US FDA. The domestic Brazilian market is generally importing drugs approved for sale in the United States and the EMEA: In the convoluted logic of international trade, a number of these products are developed in the United States, approved by the US FDA, manufactured in Brazil (under USFDA control), packaged in the United States and then resent to Brazil for public distribution.

Brazil media have recently reported claims of (a) government corruption in the selection of drugs (particular generic drugs) for domestic distribution and (b) excessive and unofficial user fees that may move a drug to the front of the Anvisa review queue. These claims have not been independently confirmed.

13.3.3   Differences Between US FDA and ANVISA

Avista has broader responsibility (including health services, regulating hospitals, and physicians) than the FDA, and it apparently lacks the budget and professional staff resources to effectively meet all of its charges. As the agency grows in experience in expertise, it will presumably follow the model of the US FDA and other international agencies and will improve effectiveness.

Note that Anvisa does not include responsibility for veterinary products and has only limited responsibility for food products. To date, it has not assumed the burden of controlling product advertising.

Anvisa has been responsible for the regulation of tobacco products since shortly after its inception, and it is much advanced over the US FDA in this area.

13.3.4   Summary

Anvisa is an emerging, maturing regulatory agency hampered by a shortage of professional resources. It is developing a series of mechanisms for effective regulation of a growing pharmaceutical industry and an emerging biologics (blood and tissue) industry.

Currently, Brazil is largely deferring to the US FDA for oversight of its growing pharmaceutical manufacturing operations.

13.3.5   Contact Information for ANVISA

Email: infovisa@anvisa.gov.br

Ombudsman's Office through phone number (61) 448-1235 or 448-1464 or through phone/fax 448-1144

13.4   CHINA

13.4.1   Description of State Food and Drug Agency (SFDA)

The State Food and Drug Agency (SFDA) of China regulates drugs, medical devices, cosmetics, food products, food-related health functions, in vitro diagnostics (IVD), biologics, and imported drug products. Interestingly, biologics are classified as drugs, and the agency has a special division devoted to health foods.

SFDA is a young agency and has been rocked with scandal. Perhaps most dramatically, the director of the SFDA, Zheng Xiaoyu, was accused of, convicted of, and executed for corruption in 2007. The agency has also suffered from charges of approving unsafe goods, including toothpaste mixed with inappropriate industrial cleansers and chemicals, tainted and expired antibiotics, and contaminated active pharmaceutical ingredients (API). While the Chinese government is taking steps to improve regulatory oversight and to avoid future problems, fundamental infrastructure factors suggest that the problems may persist. The SFDA dos not have the authority to forbid mixed-use (industrial and pharmaceutical chemicals) manufacturing facilities; SFDA personnel are underpaid, overworked, and often placed in positions beyond their skill levels; and industry has not matured sufficiently to assure primary quality control responsibility.

Most SFDA energy (and budget) has been focused on export (generally of API and of noncomplex medical devices) and import (of pharmaceuticals and biologics). As a result, the US FDA has de facto become a co-regulator and has opened a branch office in Beijing. The SFDA, in turn, has developed a specific process for approving imported drug and device products. Here, for example, is a subsection of the Initial Registration of Import Products (device):

1. The certificate issued by the government agency of the country (region) of origin to authorize the manufacturer to engage in the production and distribution of medical devices (equivalent to the business certificate or manufacturing enterprise license).

2. The qualification certificate of the applicant.

   (a) Business certificate of the applicant.

   (b) The certificate of commission given by the manufacturer to the agent for registration.

3. The certificate recognized or approved by the government of the country of Origin to authorize the products as medical devices to enter into the market of the country.

   (a) In case of any special authorization documents specified by the government of country (region) of origin for medical devices to be put into the market of the country (region) of origin, such as formal authorization documents as 510 K or PMA of the US FDA, and the CE certificate of the EU shall be submitted.

   (i) In case of one of the following circumstances:

   * That no special authorization documents are required to handle by the government of the country of Origin:

   * That in case of any change to the Products on the basis of the Products specified in the original special authorization documents, due to the difference in the partition of registration elements, no re-application is required by the government of the Country of Origin, the enterprise shall give a statement, and provide the following certificates:

1. The free sale certificate issued by the government; or

2. The certificate to the foreign government; and

3. The enterprise self-guarantee declaration in conformance with the provisions concerned of local regulations.

(b) In case of no document issued by the government of country of origin to authorize the medical devices to be put into market.

    (i) If the products shall be regulated as medical devices in the country of origin, but they have not been authorized by the government of country of origin to be put into market, the standards of the products to be registered authorized by the competent department shall be submitted; in case of products of Class II or Class III, the full-performance test report, clinical trial reports, risk analysis reports within the territory of China, and other documents necessary for the registration of import products shall be submitted, subject to which the application may be accepted, and after the acceptance the on-site inspection of the production quality system will be arranged.

    (ii) If the products shall be regulated as medical devices in the country of origin, but need not be authorized by the government of country of origin to put in the market because they are produced specifically for China, the first paragraph of this article shall be applied.

    (iii) If the products fail to be regulated as medical devices in the country of origin but the products are defined as medical devices in China in accordance with the definition of medical devices, the first paragraph of this article shall be applied.

(c) The certificates may be submitted in the form of the copy thereof, subject to the seal by the original issuing agency or the notarization by the local notarization agency.

4. The standards of the products to be registered shall apply to the provisions for the management of the medical devices standards.

(a) The methods for the implementation of "Only the Original of the Standards Sealed or Signed by the Legal Representative may be submitted":

    (i) Standards of the Products to be Registered may be sealed through the following three methods:

        * to be sealed by the Manufacturer;

        * to be sealed by the office or representative office of the Manufacturer in China;

        * to be sealed by the unit in charge of the conclusion, arrangement, drafting of the Standards of the Products to be Registered commissioned by the Manufacturer. And in the certificate of commission, it shall be clearly indicated that "the xxx Unit is commissioned to be responsible for the completion of the Standards of the Products to be Registered in China, and the Manufacturer shall be responsible for the quality of the Products".

(ii) the Definition of the Legal Representative: in accordance with the international practices, "the signature and seal of the Legal Representative" of the Manufacturer abroad may be signed and sealed by the senior official in charge of the corresponding business activities.

(b) The Standards of the Products to be Registered reviewed, codified, and recorded by SDA Standard and Technical Committee:

(c) As for the products with national standard and industrial standards, the manufacturer shall, with the implementation of the standards mentioned above, based on its own specialties, supplement and add corresponding requirements, formulate the standards of the products to be registered, and assure the safety and effectiveness of the operation of the products; if the enterprise thinks that no requirements on safety need to be added, and that the direct adoption of national standard and industrial standards as the manufacturer standards of the products to be registered is sufficient for the assurance of the safety and effectiveness of the products, the manufacturer shall submit a statement justifying that without any increase and improvement in the standard index on the basis of national standard and industrial standards, the safety and effectiveness of the products for application can be assured, declaring to bear the quality liabilities after the launching of the products and carrying the model, specification of the products. As for the products with ISO or IEC standards, the manufacturer shall convert the standards to the standards for the products to be registered.

Note the specific incorporation of ISO, IEC, and other international standards, along with the acceptance and incorporation of US FDA device approval and the CE as a standard of the SFDA.

The SFDA also has some public health responsibilities, including restaurant and food preparation organization inspections. Perhaps because of the highly centralized nature of Chinese government, a number of functions that are decentralized in the United States fall on the SFDA.

13.4.2   Pharmaceutical–Medical Device/Biologics Business in China

The China business picture is bifurcated along historical lines. Herbal products and "health foods," the basis of traditional Chinese medicine, are established businesses regulated by the SFDA. The so-called "Western" pharmaceutical–medical device–biologics industries are new, poorly regulated (probably as a result of a shortage of regulatory expertise and tradition), and relatively rare. Bridging the gap is a rapidly growing chemical industry that includes a significant pharmaceutical API component. No doubt home-grown Chinese pharmaceutical–medical device–biologics industries will grow rapidly and begin developing more new products, but currently these industries are importing formulae and replicating for domestic use, or exporting API to the United States and Europe for final product, then reimporting those products for domestic distribution.

13.4.3 Differences Between US FDA and SFDA

Many of the operational differences between US FDA and SFDA can be appropriately attributed to maturity of industry and agency; to centralization and system of government; and to historical culture. Specific functional differences include areas of responsibility: The SFDA has responsibilities overlapping (a) the Centers for Disease Control and Prevention (CDC) in the United States and (b) the US Department of Agriculture. The SFDA also has responsibility for the "healthy foods" regulation, which has no direct US equivalent.

The most dramatic difference, however, is related to the innovation of the US drug discovery, biologic development, and medical device invention industries. At this stage of its rapidly accelerating development, China is focusing on replication and support (through API manufacture) of European and American innovations. Compared to the US FDA, then, the SFDA therefore is much more involved in (a) import of finished pharmaceutical, device, and biologic products and (b) export of the raw materials that are utilized in those products.

13.4.4 Summary

The SFDA has been charged with high-level corruption, inadequate supervision, and ineffective regulation. These charges largely stem from agency challenges related to (a) the problems of a highly centralized administration in a vast and decentralized nation, (b) inadequate funding, and (c) a shortage of trained and experienced personnel in the agency.

13.4.5 Contact

State Food and Drug Administration

A38, Beilishi Road

Beijing 100810, People's Republic of China

Fax: 86-010-68310909

Email: inquires@sda.gov.cn

13.5 EUROPEAN UNION

13.5.1 Description of the European Medicines Agency (EMEA)

The European Medicines Agency is the primary regulatory body of the European Union (EU) member states, though many of these member countries also maintain their own national agencies. The EMEA defines its role as follows:

Working with the Member States and the European Commission as partners in a European medicines network, the European Medicines Agency:

- Provides independent, science-based recommendations on the quality, safety, and efficacy of medicines, as well as on more general issues relevant to public and animal health that involve medicines.

- Applies efficient and transparent evaluation procedures to help bring new medicines to the market by means of a single, EU-wide marketing authorization granted by the European Commission.

- Implements measures for continuously supervising the quality, safety, and efficacy of authorized medicines to ensure that their benefits outweigh their risks.

- Provides scientific advice and incentives to stimulate the development and improve the availability of innovative new medicines.

- Recommends safe limits for residues of veterinary medicines used in food-producing animals, for the establishment of maximum residue limits by the European Commission.

- Involves representatives of patients, healthcare professionals, and other stakeholders in its work, to facilitate dialogue on issues of common interest.

- Publishes impartial and comprehensible information about medicines and their use.

- Develops best practice for medicines evaluation and supervision in Europe, and contributes alongside the Member States and the European Commission to the harmonization of regulatory standards at the international level.

Note that the EMEA roughly parallels US FDA responsibilities, including drugs, devices, biologics, veterinary medicines, and some food products. In the years since its establishment, the EMEA has obtained a strong and positive scientific reputation, along with a reputation for reasonable efficiency.

The EMEA incorporates six scientific committees that generally parallel the research role of the US National Institutes of Health: Medical Products for Human Use (CHMP), Medical Products for Veterinary Use (CVMP), Orphan Medical Products (COMP), Herbal Medical Products (HMPC), Pediatric Committee (PDCO), and the Committee for Advanced Therapies (CAT). Unlike the organizational scheme of the US FDA, these target population centers incorporate all relevant therapies: pharmaceutical, device, and biologics.

13.5.2 Pharmaceutical–Medical Device–Biologics Business in the European Union

The EU countries have a strong history of product development: Germany has long been the center of pharmaceutical development; France and its Pasteur Institute have originated many biologic products; the United Kingdom, the Scandinavian Countries, and the Netherlands originated many of the medical device inventions that dominate today's medical market. Today the EMEA regulates a business opportunity second only to the United States (and, as the EU continues to expand, challenging that predominance), and the EU countries represent a continuing center for new product development, manufacture, and innovation.

As the pharmaceutical, medical device, and biologics industries have become increasingly global, the EMEA and US FDA have cooperated to regulate international companies and their products. Many drugs and devices are jointly registered with both agencies (see Chapter 14 on concurrent registration for cost-containing recommendations). In addition, many of the employees of international companies find themselves stationed in alternating regions, assigned wherever their talents are needed; as a result, regulatory professionals in major organizations are generally cross trained in US FDA and EMEA requirements and have developed harmonization strategies to cope with relatively minor differences.

Over the next decade, increased EMEA and US FDA cooperation, driven by increased internationalization of the industry, are geared to continue the trend toward globalization of the pharmaceutical, medical device, and biologics industries.

13.5.3   Differences Between USFDA and EMEA

The remaining differences between EMEA and US FDA fall into three general categories: confederate structure, reliance on the device CE Mark, and general regulatory philosophy.

The United States is dominated by a federal government: a strong, central body with predominant control in most areas over individual state responsibilities. Pennsylvania, for example, has long-standing regulations relating to baked goods. But since trade crosses state borders, the US FDA trumps those requirements for most related products. For all practical purposes, the US FDA is the only significant regulator of pharmaceutical, medical device, and biologics products in the United States.

The European Union, on the other hand, is a confederation of sovereign countries. While the EMEA is the common body for the regulation of pharmaceutical, medical device, and biologics products within that confederation, each individual member country may establish (or may have previously established) its own regulatory agency. These individual agencies can interpret general EMEA rules, may differ in their enforcement, and, in certain conditions, may supplement with their own guidelines and regulations. This decentralization, coupled with the confederate nature of the EU, often results in EMEA regulations that are compromises and composites. The result has generally been positive (resulting in a broad scientific consensus), but may prove alien to organizations more used to the more rigid power position of the US FDA.

Another difference between US FDA and the EMEA is the reliance on the CE Mark. The CE Mark is an EU government program designed to assure the safety of any product sold in the European Union. Products are independently tested for safety, and awarded the mark, prior to sale. The program uses standards not unlike voluntary testing programs in the United States, but is mandatory and government controlled.

Because all medical devices are subject to the CE Mark program, the EMEA can focus its medical device review attention on product efficacy (accept in the case of high risk implanted devices, for which additional safety testing beyond the CE Mark is generally required). The current (2010) US FDA medical device review procedure often relies on predicate device citation for evidence of efficacy and focuses on safety testing; the EMEA may be able to begin its review with CE Mark evidence of safety and focus its review on the effectiveness of the device.

Finally, there is a historical and cultural difference between the EMEA and the US FDA. The US FDA has traditionally seen itself as obstructionistic: Its defined role is that of a barrier, protecting public health and safety from fraudulent products, unsafe devices, and untested therapies. The European attitude is much more cooperation-based, emphasizing the agency's role in helping to bring products and therapies to the population it serves. These philosophical differences may not always result in significantly different outcomes, but they are reflected in the attitudes of the agencies and their willingness to cooperate with industry. The EMEA often functions as a partner, offering guidance and suggestions to achieve compliance, while all too often the US FDA seems to assume the role of a police force, suspicious of all outsiders.

13.5.4 Summary

The EMEA is a modern, efficient agency closely cooperating with the US FDA and increasingly coordinating activities. While interpretations and some differences may exist between member states (see Sections 13.6 and 13.7), the organization has significantly streamlined cost containment within the EU and also for outside organizations desiring to sell within the EU.

13.5.5 Contact

European Medicines Agency

7 Westferry Circus

Canary Wharf

London E14 4HB, United Kingdom

Telephone switchboard: +44 (0)20 7418 8400

Web site: www.ema.europa.eu

13.6 FRANCE

13.6.1 Description of Agence Française de Sécurité Santaire des Produits de Santé (AFSSAPS)

Description of Agence Francaise de Sécurité Santaire des Produits de Santé (AFSSAPS) is a well-regarded, well-established national regulatory body closely with the EMEA to control the French pharmaceutical, medical device, and biologics industries. Although cosmetics and alternate medicine products are food products, they do not fall within the purview of AFSSAPS.

France has a highly centralized government with strong control authority. Production sites must be pre-licensed as GMP compliant; in-country developed and important products must submit appropriate documentation (generally including clinical results) for pre-sale review. EMEA-approved products may be distributed within France, but many French companies co-submit regulatory approval application to both EMEA and AFSSAPS to maximize acceptance.

13.6.2 Pharmaceutical/Devices/Biologics Business in France

France has a strong and long history of product development, including the development of vaccines and biologics (centered at the Pasteur Institute) and the development of pharmaceutical products in private companies along the Swiss and German border regions. The medical device industry in France is somewhat less active, though still more advanced than many countries.

Because of cultural and governmental requirements forcing dominance of French language and tradition, there seems to be less cross-national fertilization of personnel than in other European countries. Where many Europeans relocate readily to accept new positions, French citizens often refuse to do so. The result is a French industry with many non-French workers, but few French researchers in outside positions.

13.6.3 Differences Between USFDA and AFSSAPS

The major difference between the regulatory environment in the United States and in France is the two-tier French system resulting from the EMEA. While careful steps are taken to avoid conflicting requirements and to minimize redundancy, there are inevitable problems for French companies registering products for sale throughout the EU and globally.

Other differences include scope of responsibility; attitude; and balance. A significant portion of US FDA resources are spent in areas falling outside the AFSSAPS: food products, import (largely an EMEA function), and advertising. The AFSSAPS is therefore able to more tightly focus its responsibilities. This focus is sharpened by a strong tradition of very well qualified (and appropriately compensated) professional and scientific staff.

As described previously, the US FDA has a largely adversarial relationship with industry. The AFSSAPS, on the other hand, is established to assist product developers (often university or institute related) with the approval process. Cooperation between AFSSAPS and industry is well established.

Finally, in the delicate balance between public access to therapies and safety protection of that public, the US FDA falls strongly on the safety side. The French AFSSAPS describes its function as assuring that medications are available to everyone. The result is greater French price pressure but a lesser degree of regulatory control.

13.6.4 Summary

The AFSSAPS is a well-operated, modern and largely corruption free regulatory body populated by well-qualified scientists and staff. It coordinates effectively with EMEA, often from a superior position. The agency relies heavily on industry self-regulation (using requirements documents such as the CGMP).

13.6.5 Contact

143-147 Blvd Anatole, France

93285 Saint-Denis Cedex France

Telephone: +33 155 87 3000

Fax: +33 155 87 3172

www.afssaps.fr

13.7 GERMANY

13.7.1 Description of Federal Institute for Drugs and Medical Devices (Bundesinstitut FÜR Arzneimittel und Medizinprodukte, BfArM

The BfArM shares with AFSSAPS (France) and other EU member country agencies a duality of responsibility, overlapping and coordinating with the EMEA. Significant cultural differences exist, however. Where the French seem to be continuously struggling to assume a predominant role, the BfArM positions itself as a separate but equal partner in the regulation of German pharmaceuticals, medical devices, and biologics. The Mission Statement of the agency clearly strikes this note:

BfArM Mission Statement

Protection of human health is our highest goal. We therefore strive together towards guaranteeing the best possible provision of medicinal products and medical devices to the general public as well as towards preventing the abuse of narcotic drugs.

Our attention is focused on the quality, efficacy, and safety of medicinal products as well as on the implementation of measures to monitor the legal trade in narcotic drugs and their precursors. Continuous effort and workflow streamlining are necessary if the high standards of quality in our work are to be maintained. This goal is supported by experimental research in fields related to BfArM's areas of responsibility. We will enter into a constructive dialogue with all concerned and will increase the transparency of our actions by means of an objective and unbiased information policy.

We fulfill our responsibility for protecting human health without neglecting the importance of medicinal products and medical devices as economic goods. Industry is entitled to a modern and internationally competitive partner with regard to the licensing, registration, and risk monitoring of their products. Only with this approach can we position and successfully assert ourselves as a progressive and competitive institution within and beyond Europe. We confidently seek cooperative networking and constructive competition with other European licensing authorities.

A well-trained and motivated staff, working together as a team, is fundamental to the fulfillment of our duties. We therefore promote basic, further, and advanced training; equal opportunity at all levels; and the integration of family and career.

Together, we all wish to actively fulfill this mission statement, presenting our achievements with confidence, proud of our past performance, and eagerly awaiting the new challenges to come.

The BfArM is a highly structured organization, with more specific and detailed guidelines and requirements than most international regulatory agencies. Not surprisingly, though, the BfArM enjoys an excellent reputation for scientific expertise, for efficiency, and for diligence. The agency is generally considered corruption-free and is a model for many other nations.

The BfArM focuses on drugs (with a special center for narcotics), devices, and biologics and does not have responsibility for foods or cosmetics.

13.7.2 Pharmaceutical–Medical Devices–Biologics Business in Germany

The drug industry effectively began in Germany, and German companies (now often global) have dominated ever since. Many medical devices and device systems also are of German origin and modern manufacture. The vaccine and biologics industries are of lesser importance, but still rank highly on the world stage. Germany has a very strong university system that has produced an excellent science base feeding discoveries to large in emerging companies able to develop and commercialize.

The German economy is among the world's strongest, and the business climate is highly supportive. The use of the so-called foreign workers program has provided an employment buffer, and a strong investment capital system has promoted industrial development. The government is supportive, noncorrupt, and highly centralized.

13.7.3 Differences Between US FDA and BfArM

The BfArM operates very much like the US FDA, with two fundamental differences. First, the two-tier nature of a sovereign nation's regulatory body (BfArM) operating in cooperation with a treaty-liked regulatory agency (The EU's EMEA) is a situation not paralleled in the United States. The impact is largely felt with imported products, where EMEA approval may restrict BfArM from exercising primary approval control over a drug, biologic, or medical device.

Second, the two agencies differ in scope. The BfArM does not regulate cosmetic products, food products, or advertising. This focus allows the agency to more tightly concentrate on the areas and products that are arguably most directly related to public health and safety. On the other hand, the restriction forces the BfArM to more closely coordinate with other agencies and is more likely to result in the kinds of coordination conflicts that have haunted US FDA and US Department of Agriculture (each responsible for different areas of food regulation) other the years.

13.7.4 Summary

The BfArM is a modern, scandal-free, professional organization functioning effectively in a country that is one of the world's leaders in the development of drug and medical devices (and, to a lesser degree, of biologics). Working closely with the EMEA, the BfArM has developed and enforced clear guidelines and requirements, cooperating closely with a strong discovery, development, and manufacturing industry.

13.7.5 Contact

Bundesinstitut für Arzneimittel und Medizinprodukte

Kurt-Georg-Kiesinger-Allee 3

D-53175 Bonn, Germany

Telephone: +49 (0)228 99-307-0
Telefax: +49 (0)228 99-307-5207

Email: poststelle@bfarm.de

13.8 INDIA

13.8.1 Description of Central Drug Standard Control Organization (CDSCO)

The Central Drugs Standard Control Organization (CDSCO) of India is an over-worked, underfunded agency lacking in sufficient scientific expertise. It operates in cooperation with the State Drug Control Organization, and it concentrates largely on Global Clinical Trials and on import and export of drugs and active pharmaceutical ingredients (API).

CDSCO has responsibility for pharmaceutical products, biologics, cosmetics, and some limited medical devices. Perhaps uniquely, India's CDSCO has a special program to control clinical trial drugs. Coupled with a defined process for approval human drug trials, the CDSCO seems to be primarily operating to support international drug development and manufacturing, as much concerned with growing the India economy as with protecting the public health and safety within India.

Coordination with state agencies is a major issue for CDSCO, with a number of overlapping areas of responsibility. See Figure 13.1.

CDSCO has been relatively scandal-free in recent years, though its chronic funding problems suggest that the agency may not be equipped to fully evaluate all of the growing number of submissions and applications within its areas of concern. Joint programs with WHO, in effect adopting WHO Good Manufacturing Practice guidelines, may help speed the review process.

13.8.2 Pharmaceutical–Medical Device/Biologics Business in India

India enjoys a large and thriving pharmaceutical and biologics industry, with a less developed medical device operation. While drug discovering and biologics development activities are increasing, currently the business base is built upon the manu-

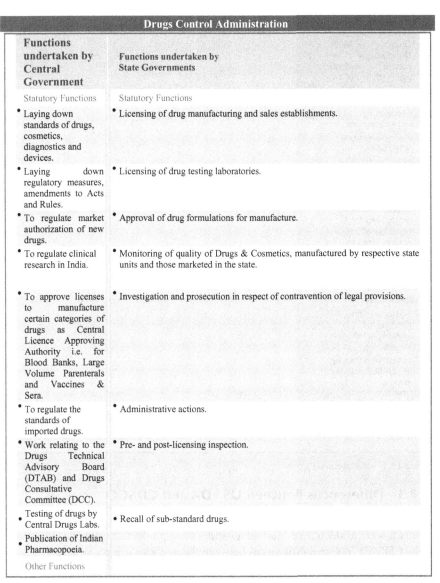

Drugs Control Administration	
Functions undertaken by Central Government	**Functions undertaken by State Governments**
Statutory Functions	Statutory Functions
• Laying down standards of drugs, cosmetics, diagnostics and devices.	• Licensing of drug manufacturing and sales establishments.
• Laying down regulatory measures, amendments to Acts and Rules.	• Licensing of drug testing laboratories.
• To regulate market authorization of new drugs.	• Approval of drug formulations for manufacture.
• To regulate clinical research in India.	• Monitoring of quality of Drugs & Cosmetics, manufactured by respective state units and those marketed in the state.
• To approve licenses to manufacture certain categories of drugs as Central Licence Approving Authority i.e. for Blood Banks, Large Volume Parenterals and Vaccines & Sera.	• Investigation and prosecution in respect of contravention of legal provisions.
• To regulate the standards of imported drugs.	• Administrative actions.
• Work relating to the Drugs Technical Advisory Board (DTAB) and Drugs Consultative Committee (DCC).	• Pre- and post-licensing inspection.
• Testing of drugs by Central Drugs Labs.	• Recall of sub-standard drugs.
• Publication of Indian Pharmacopoeia.	
Other Functions	

Figure 13.1

facture of generic drugs, the production of API, and the recruitment and operation of clinical trials.

The relatively decentralization of India, coupled with the phenomenal economic growth of recent years, has placed the expansion of the pharmaceutical businesses well ahead of efforts at meaningful regulation. CDSCO is constantly playing catch up, relying on whistle blower programs and extra-national organizations like the US FDA and WHO in lieu of sufficient in-house expertise and investigators to exercise real regulatory control.

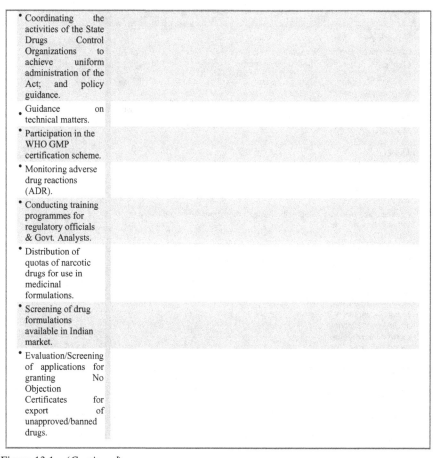

* Coordinating the activities of the State Drugs Control Organizations to achieve uniform administration of the Act; and policy guidance.
* Guidance on technical matters.
* Participation in the WHO GMP certification scheme.
* Monitoring adverse drug reactions (ADR).
* Conducting training programmes for regulatory officials & Govt. Analysts.
* Distribution of quotas of narcotic drugs for use in medicinal formulations.
* Screening of drug formulations available in Indian market.
* Evaluation/Screening of applications for granting No Objection Certificates for export of unapproved/banned drugs.

Figure 13.1 (*Continued*)

13.8.3 Differences Between US FDA and CDSCO

The US FDA includes control of all medical devices, veterinary pharmaceuticals, (now) tobacco products, and some advertising; these products are outside the purview of the CDSCO. The real differences between the agencies are not structural or even budgetary, however; they are clearly attitudinal.

The US FDA operates as a barrier control excesses of industry, protecting the public from untested or undertested and control substances and devices. In a real sense the US FDA is responsible for policing the pharmaceutical, biologics, and device industries.

The CDSCO seems to be closer to a Chamber of Commerce than to a barrier organization. More funds and more energy are directed toward helping to grow the industry than toward keeping that industry in check.

13.8.4 Summary

India has a modern regulatory agency and an appropriate series of regulations and guidelines. Lacking is (a) the funding to build a strong and growing scientific team to enforce those laws and (b) the will to control a very important national industry focusing on generic manufacture, API manufacture, and clinical trials. These functions are all oriented toward export, while internal pharmaceutical development is split between national and state agencies with some overlapping responsibilities.

13.8.5   Contact

Central Drugs Standard Control Organization

Directorate General of Health Services

Ministry of Health and Family Welfare

Government of India

FDA Bhavan, ITO

Kotla Road

New Delhi 110002, India

Phone: 91-11-23236965 / 23236975

Fax: 91-11-23236973

13.9   ISRAEL

13.9.1   Description of Ministry of Health (IMOH)

The Israel Ministry of Health (IMOH) regulates pharmaceuticals, biologics, and medical devices within Israel. The Israeli population and hence market, however, as so small that the IMOH would not normally command a spot on this limited list of the most active regulatory agencies and largest industrial players. However, Israel has two characteristics of particular interest. First, despite its small size, Israel is the global leader in the development of new medical devices. This predominant development position is in part a result of the immigration of a large engineering population from the old Soviet Union at the end of the cold war, and in part a result of a focus program supported by the Israeli Office of the Chief Scientist, which funds medical device entrepreneurs.

Second, Israel is representative of the large number of small national that have in effect outsourced regulatory responsibility to the larger countries. This strategy in effect requires an importer to provide evidence that other major regulatory body has approved a product, and then simply reviews that regulatory report. Consider, for example, this section from the medical device regulations of the Israel:

> Medical Devices, including biologics, must be registered with Israel's Ministry of Health (IMOH) before they can be sold in the country. Companies wishing to export medical equipment or devices to Israel must have a local Israeli agent or distributor who should request a pre-marketing approval from the IMOH. The request should be accompanied by one of the following documents: the US Food and Drug Administration (FDA) 510(k), or Pre-Market Approval (PMA). Biological devices fall under medical device classification and require FDA's

Center of Biologics certificate. In most cases CE and Canadian documentation are also acceptable by IMOH.

If a product is approved by the US FDA, it will be registered by the MOH with no further testing. However, electromedical devices must be tested at the Standard Institute of Israel (SII) for compliance with the Israeli system. The SII does not accept certifications from other countries.

For any imported medical device the Israeli importer/agent must submit a registration application to MOH Department of Medical Devices. The application should include (if available) a certificate issued by a competent authority of one of the following countries: Australia, Canada, European Community (CE) Member States (MSs), Japan, or the United States of America.

The IMOH, limited in resources, has in effect agreed to accept evaluation and certification from other major regulators.

13.9.2 Pharmaceutical–Medical Devices–Biologics Business in Israel

The Israeli pharmaceutical industry is largely limited to discovery (centered in universities) and generic manufacturing (often directed from Israel and conducted globally, as in the TEVA model). Similarly, biologics and device industries tend to development or discover and to license production abroad. Israel has, in effect, perfected the process of licensing intellectual property.

There is one interesting area of clinical research developed in Israel. Because the country has such a large percentage of immigrants (without wandering into a major political and/or biblical debate, arguably a significant portion of the population is non-native), researchers as Ben Gurion University have realized that there are residents who have been exposed to a vast number of different diseases, including plague, malaria, dengue, ebola, smallpox, and so on. Their immune systems make excellent test laboratories for new vaccine development. These researchers have therefore launched a globally significant (in importance rather than numbers) series of clinical studies of newly perfect vaccines.

The major business development in the pharmaceutical, device, and biologics industries in Israel is, of course, in the development of new medical devices. A number of strategic industrial parks, private and government investment funding, an abundance of scientists and engineers, and a long history of wars and war injuries have led to a thriving industry that generally registers its output in the United States (under USFDA 510(k) and PMA provisions) and then licenses products to US companies for manufacture and/or distribution.

13.9.3 Differences Between USFDA and IMOH

The IMOH has broad responsibilities overlapping US FDA, CDC, and NIH. This combination of tasks allows some greater direction of industry toward national health needs; a greater resource in scientific expertise; and a broader picture of international cooperation. The major difference between US FDA and IMOH is, again, one of attitude. IMOH is charged with encouraging and assisting the industries it regulates, while USFDA has a much more skeptical police mentality.

That attitudinal difference is also obvious in the two regulatory agencies' position regarding coordinating and harmonization with international bodies. The IMOH all but requires registration with one of the major national agencies (United States, Japan, EMEA, etc.), while the United States requires independent and separate submission regardless of other approvals. While on the surface this policy would seem to assure greater safety with US-sold products, Israel's experience suggests that a cross-acceptance does not compromise safety while permitting a significant savings or redirection of funding.

13.9.4 Summary

Israel stands as the leader in new medical device invention, and it also serves as a model of cooperation with other global and national regulatory agencies. That cooperation and co-opting of other regulatory agency reviews is a common and successful strategy of other small countries around the world.

13.9.5 Contact

Ministry of Health

2 Ben Tabai St.

Jerusalem, Israel 91010

972-2-6705705

972-2-5681200

Email: pniot@moh.health.gov.il

13.10 JAPAN

13.10.1 Description of Pharmaceuticals and Medical Devices Agency (PMDA)

The PMDA is a modern, efficient regulatory agency with a well-designed budget, high-level professional staff, and a tradition of effective and corruption free protection of the Japanese public health and safety. It performs these responsibilities in close cooperation with industry, and it achieves a near-ideal balance between safety and access to health-care products.

PMDA has primary responsibility for oversight of the pharmaceutical, medical device, and biologics industries; cosmetics, foods, and veterinary products are regulated separately. The PMDA approves new products for internal Japanese distribution and for export; reviews manufacturing facilities; monitors use and application; develops and promulgates standards; promotes the public health; and enforces regulations. Not surprisingly, the PMDA operates in much the same manner as the US FDA, on which it was modeled.

13.10.2   Pharmaceutical–Medical Devices–Biologics Business in Japan

While its official role is centered on the public health and safety, the PMDA maintains close industry ties and seems to be heavily involved in encouraging and cooperating with Japanese industry. That industry is a leader in all aspects of the field: New pharmaceutical products are discovered, developed, and manufactured; biologics are purified, tested, and developed; and medical devices are designed, improved, and manufactured.

It is sometimes difficult for a non-Japanese company to effectively operate in Japan, largely due to cultural and linguistic complications. The PMDA has generally been a helpful partner to US and European companies seeking to enter the Japanese market with unique products, though a separate registration and review is necessary: Like the United States, Japan does not automatically accept the approval of a product from another regulatory agency.

13.10.3   Differences Between US FDA and PMDA

The PMDA has it roots in the forced government reorganization by occupying US troops at the conclusion of the Second World War, and hence it is very similar to the US FDA in structure and purpose. The PMDA has a narrow area of responsibility (as described above), and functionally it seems much more cooperative (rather than obstructionistic) than the US FDA.

Japan has been a very active player in international harmonization efforts, working toward international Good Manufacturing Practices and Good Laboratory Practices. The PMDA has played a leading role in these discussions. Because of Japan's important position as an exporter of drugs, biologics, and medical devices, standardized regulations are generally viewed as valuable tools of business development.

13.10.4   Summary

In many ways Japan is a model of regulatory efficiency and industry cooperation. The PMDA is a leading regulatory agency promoting and protecting national health and safety. While some non-Japanese companies may complain of barriers to import, the PMDA's reputation for technically accomplished, effectively funded, professionally managed efficiency is strong.

13.10.5   Contact

Pharmaceuticals and Medical Devices Agency

Shin-Kasumigaseki Building

3-3-2 Kasumigaseki

Chiyoda-ku, Tokyo 100-0013 Japan

Telephone: +81-3-3506-9456

Fax: +81-3-3506-9572

Email: info.pmda.f10@pmda.go.jp

13.11   KOREA (SOUTH)

13.11.1   Description of Korea Food and Drug Administration (KDFA)

The Korean Food and Drug Administration (KDFA) is a modern, efficient regulatory agency somewhat handicapped by budgetary restrictions and a shortage of expert personnel. Despite these minor problems, the agency has a history of effectively protecting public health and safety while encouraging and promoting South Korean pharmaceutical, medical device, and biologics industries. The KDFA is responsible for cosmetics and foods as well as drugs, medical devices, vaccines, and biologicals, and it focuses on both a growing in-country industry and the important of products for domestic consumption.

In 2009 the KDFA underwent a massive reorganization, including the consolidation of 114 divisions to 98; the addition of a Criminal investigation Office and a Foreign Inspection Division; the establishment of a National Institute of Food and Drug Safety Evaluation; and an inspection decentralization, with many functions transferred to city and provincial governments. While a full evaluation of the success of this reorganization is still pending, preliminary results suggest an improvement in regulatory control within existing budgets, along with a more efficient system of new product review and approval.

13.11.2   Pharmaceutical–Medical Devices–Biologics Business in South Korea

The Republic of Korea is working to promote its pharmaceutical, biologics, and medical device industries. Thus far the greatest successes have been in the production of active pharmaceutical ingredients, in generic drug manufacture (largely for domestic use), and in the production of components for medical devices. There is, however, a strong discovery base that is beginning to result in new products and patents. The KDFA, particularly under its new reorganization, is actively helping to promote these industries.

South Korea remains a major contract manufacturer of disposable medical products and components for complex medical devices. These industries, utilizing molding, extrusion, and other technologies, are beginning to expand their capabilities as segments focus exclusively on the medical device marketplace.

The Republic of Korea is also beginning to export generic drug products for sales and distribution in other parts of Asia, including Taiwan and Viet Nam.

13.11.3   Differences Between US FDA and KFDA

The US FDA and KFDA are very similar in organization (after the Korean reorganization of 2009), philosophy, and regulatory standards. This similarity is not accidental: The two countries are closely linked in recent history and as trading partners, making regulatory cooperation a very positive attribute.

The KFDA is, or course, much smaller in size, and it relies more heavily on local city and provincial investigators and inspectors than does the US FDA. But informal harmonization efforts have been effective: while there is no imminent likelihood of cross registration, products approved by the United States are generally acceptable to the KFDA, and Korean products have not been the subject of major skepticism by the US FDA.

13.11.4 Summary

The KFDA is a modern, increasingly efficient national regulatory body coordinating closely with US FDA. A recent reorganization has brought the two agencies closer into alignment. Korea plans to expand their industries, and exports have resulted in efforts to keep the KDFA sufficiently funded, well-staffed with qualified experts, and up to date in standards and interpretations.

13.11.5 Contact

194 Tongiro

Eunpyeoung-gu

Seoul 122-704, Republic of Korea

Email: kdfa@kdfa@go.kr

13.12 SWITZERLAND

13.12.1 Description of Swissmedic

Swissmedic is the Swiss agency for therapeutic products, including pharmaceuticals, medical devices, and biologics. The agency is divided into seven product groups: human medicines, herbals, veterinary products, narcotics, blood products, medical devices, and transplants. Switzerland has a long history of development and manufacture of pharmaceutical products, coordinating closely with operations in Germany and France. In fact the Swiss center for pharmaceutical operations, Basel, is located at the junction of the three countries, with overlapping employees and occasional facilities. Despite these close ties, however, Switzerland is not a member of the EU and hence not subject to EMEA oversight. Despite this separation, however, Switzerland coordinates closely with international regulatory agencies (see below), working with EMEA, US FDA, and other authorities.

Swissmedic is a professional, well regarded agency with sufficient funding and resources to perform its tasks effectively. It has attracted a high professional scientific staff, well regarded domestically and internationally.

13.12.2 Pharmaceutical–Medical Devices–Biologics Business in Switzerland

The pharmaceutical industry in Switzerland (and, to a lesser but still significant degree, the devices and biologics industries) are well established, well capitalized, and effectively managed in close cooperation with Swissmedic. In fact, Swissmedic defines its primary task as one of collaboration with industry and with other regulatory bodies:

> In May 2008, the Agency Council decided upon a concept for Swissmedic's national and international collaboration with the relevant stakeholders.
>
> An important principle of the collaboration is the involvement of all external stakeholders, with their frequently diverging interests, in the activities of Swissmedic.
>
> To achieve this, transparency plays a major role: It is necessary for processes and decisions to be auditable externally.
>
> Implementing the objectives established within the concept calls for communication that is active, reactive, and also passive and that is appropriate for the various target groups.
>
> Collaboration is based on a relationship that creates and maintains trust and that promotes mutual understanding.
>
> Efficient communication with the various stakeholders, with a view to improving mutual comprehension, information exchange and the results thus obtained, is an aspect that is at the foreground of the concept.

In this connection, stakeholders are those persons or groups that are concerned either by Swissmedic's legally mandated activities or by the measures resulting thereof, or who have legal entitlements regarding Swissmedic's activities.

This concept of collaboration leads to close cooperation and coordination, often lead and initiated by the professional staff of Swissmedic. The effect has been a continuing leader role for a relatively small and self-contained nation and its regulatory agency. See Figure 13.2.

13.12.3 Differences Between US FDA and Swissmedic

There are two major differences between US FDA and Swissmedic: organizational and attitudinal. Organizationally Swissmedic has established two divisions—narcotics and transplants—that have not received independent focus within the US FDA and that overlap other US federal agencies (in particular the Drug Enforcement Agency, DEA, with some separate responsibility for narcotics products).

The spirit of collaboration that forms the foundation of Swissmedic distinguishes the agency from the protectionistic attitude of the US FDA. The Swiss pendulum is generally in the "access" quadrant, while the US FDA focuses largely on safety. As a result, US FDA spends most of its energy and budget on policing rather that cooperating with industry.

13.12.4 Summary

In many ways, Swissmedic represents a "new and improved" model of regulation of the pharmaceutical, medical device, and biologics industries, emphasizing collaboration, professionalism, and an organizational schema incorporating herbal and supplemental products, transplantations, and other cutting-edge technologies.

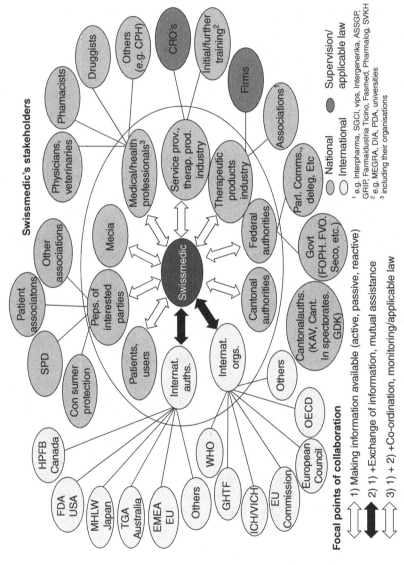

Swissmedic's stakeholders

CRO's

Druggists

Others (e.g. CPH)

Initial/further training[2]

Pharmacists

Firms

Physicians, veterinaries

Medical/health professionals[3]

Service prov., therap. prod. industry

Associations[1]

Therapeutic products industry

Other associations

Mecia

Parl. Comms., deleg, Etc

Patient associatons

Peps. of interested parties

Swissmedic

Federal authorities

SPD

Con sumer protection

Patients, users

Internat. auths.

Govt (FOPH, FVO, Seco, etc.)

Internat. orgs.

Cantonal authorities

Cantonalauths. (KAV, Cant. In spectorates. GDK)

Others

OECD

HPFB Canada

WHO

FDA USA

MHLW Japan

GHTF

European Council

TGA Australia

(ICH/VICH)

EMEA EU

Others

EU Commission

National
International

Supervision/
applicable law

[1] e.g. Interpharma, SGCI, vips, Intergenerika, ASSGP, GRIP, Farmaidustria Ticino, Fasmed, Pharmalog, SVKH
[2] e.g. MEGRA, DIA, PDA, universities
[3] including their organisations

Focal points of collaboration

1) Making information available (active, passive, reactive)

2) 1) +Exchange of information, mutual assistance

3) 1) + 2) +Co-ordination, monitoring/applicable law

Figure 13.2 Swissmedic's stakeholders map

13.12.5   Contact

Swissmedic

Swiss Agency for Therapeutic Products

Hallerstrasse 7

CH-3000 Bern 9, Switzerland

Phone: +41 31 322 02 11

Fax: +41 31 322 02 12

13.13   UNITED KINGDOM

13.13.1   Description of Medicines and Health-Care Products Regulatory Agency (MHRA)

MHRA is a modern, professional agency working in close cooperation with the EMEA (the United Kingdom is a member of the European Union). The agency is adequately funded and has a reputation and responsibility that attracts a professional scientific staff of appropriate high repute.

MHRA regulates medicines, medical devices, advanced therapy medical products such as radiological products, nanotechnology, and blood products. In addition to its central office (see Contact, Section 13.3.5), the agency has regional offices actively involved in inspection and investigation of developmental and manufacturing facilities.

13.13.2   Pharmaceutical–Medical Devices–Biologics Business in the United Kingdom

The UK enjoys a large and active pharmaceutical industry; and innovative and well-regarded medical devices industry; and a somewhat more limited but successfully focused biologics industry. These industries supply the domestic market; are primary suppliers to the old Commonwealth; and distributed widely within the EU (and to some degree within the United States).

While most UK pharmaceutical companies are likely to be global in their manufacturing and distribution systems, the majority of discovery is connected to researchers at UK universities and most of the product development activities are focused in the United Kingdom. Similarly, device and biologics companies are generally conducting their research and development activities in the United Kingdom.

13.13.3   Differences Between US FDA and MHRA

Unlike the US FDA, MHRA does not share responsibility for food products. Interestingly, veterinary products and human medicines are coordinated through the same "medicines" division, perhaps an improvement over the US FDA's separation policy.

The major difference between US FDA and MHRA is the two-tier nature of the UK system, described above under France and Germany (Sections 13.6 and 13.7). UK companies seeking to sell with the EU are subject to both MHRA and EMEA regulation, making close coordination critically important.

While the MHRA has, at least on paper, more of the industry cooperation function than does the US FDA, many UK company executives express the same frustrations with the agency as do US FDA-regulated companies. Either officially or unofficially, both agencies seem to have "barrier mentalities," emphasizing protection of the public from dangerous drugs over their roles of helping to assure public access to valuable therapies.

13.13.4   Summary

The MHR is a professional, well-respected agency dedicated to "ensuring that medicines and medical devices work and are acceptably safe." It performs this task effectively in close cooperation with the EMEA and in coordination with the US FDA and other national regulatory agencies.

13.13.5   Contact

10-2 Market Towers

1 Nine Elms Lane

London SW8 5NQ, United Kingdom

Tel: 020 7084 2000 (weekdays 0900–1700)

Tel: 020 7210 3000 (other times)

Fax: 020 7084 2353

Email: info@mhra.gsi.gov.uk

13.13.6   Cost Containment

Many of the same cost-containment strategies identified in this text are directly applicable to international regulatory agencies. The concept of utilizing a credible independent audit, for example, will prove effective in all the countries described. Similarly, the use of electronic submission is rapidly gaining universal favor, particularly as newly emerging agencies leapfrog over less productive paper technologies and move directly to electronic communications. Finally, the concept of risk assessment to focus regulatory attention seems to be universal, particularly because most regulatory agencies are more interested to assuring public access to therapies and the minor compromise of safety goals.

Other strategies are less universally accepted. Quality by Design (QbD) is rapidly emerging in Australia, the EU countries, and Switzerland, but has little traction elsewhere. Clarifying definitions similarly will prove effective in the EU but has little value in other regions. Outsourcing is a strategy of Europe but has no caught

TABLE 13.1 International Regulatory Agencies and Regulation Procedures

Nation	Agency	Operational Definitions	Pre-Audits	Quality by Design	Outsourcing	Electronic Solutions	EMEA	Visits	Risk
United States	US FDA	x	x	x	x	x	x	x	x
Australia	TGA	x	x	x		x	x	x	x
Brazil	Anvisa	x	x			x	x	x	x
China	SFDA	x	x			x		x	x
EU	EMEA		x	x	x	x	NA		x
France	AFSSAPS	x	x	x		x	NA		x
Germany	BfArM	x	x	x	x	x	NA		x
India	CDSCO		x			x		x	x
Israel	IMOH		x			x			x
Japan	PMDA		x	x		x	x		x
Korea (South)	KFDA	x	x	x		x		x	x
Switzerland	Swissmed		x	x		x	x		x
United Kingdom	MHRA	x	x	x	x	x	NA		x

NA, not available.

on elsewhere. And suggestions for streamlining US FDA visits have the greatest value, obviously, in those countries where US FDA visits are most common and in which other regulatory agencies do not follow the same procedures.

As a final note, the pharmaceutical industry in particular and the biologics and device industries to lesser degrees are global in scope. Discovery, development, and manufacturing may be divided among a variety of countries. Similarly, a company and product may end up regulated by a variety of different agencies. Cost containment in the broadest sense, along with product cost control for product end users, is largely dependent upon the degree to which these various regulatory agencies collaborate to avoid unnecessary duplication and redundancy. See Table 13.1.

CHAPTER 14

COST-CONTAINED REGULATORY COMPLIANCE

Contributing author: Dr. Ron Fuqua

The accountability of medical device and drug manufacturers has been the subject of substantial debate and analysis. The increased interest in accountability, or cost-contained regulatory compliance, has been attributed to a number of factors, including rapid growth of the sectors and their role as major economic actors, increased influence of NGOs such as WHO, ISO, OECD, and ICH in shaping public policy, and the "crisis of legitimacy" stemming from highly publicized scandals in a variety of sectors. Several strategies have been developed for accomplishing cost-contained regulatory compliance including: Operational Definitions, Pre-Audits, Quality by Design, Outsourcing, Electronic Submissions, and EMEA Overlap.

The rising interest in cost-contained regulatory compliance has been accompanied by increased interest in addressing accountability issues through self-regulation. Both in the United States and in other countries, a variety of regulatory programs have been created. These efforts have involved the establishment and promulgation of standards for ethical behavior by which member or rated organizations are expected to be governed. Several nongovernmental organizations (NGOs) are playing the principal role in these efforts.

The World Health Organization (WHO) is the directing and coordinating authority for health within the United Nations system and is responsible for providing leadership on global health matters, shaping the health research agenda, setting norms and standards, articulating evidence-based policy options, providing technical support to countries, and monitoring and assessing health trends. In the twenty-first century, health is a shared responsibility, involving equitable access to essential care and collective defense against transnational threats. The WHO agenda includes six action points:

1. *Promoting Development.* Health has achieved unprecedented prominence as a key driver of socioeconomic progress, and more resources than ever are being invested in health. However, poverty continues to contribute to poor health, and poor health anchors large populations in poverty. For the WHO, health development is directed by the ethical principle of equity: Access to

Cost-Contained Regulatory Compliance: For the Pharmaceutical, Biologics, and Medical Device Industries, First Edition. Sandy Weinberg.
© 2011 John Wiley & Sons, Inc. Published 2011 by John Wiley & Sons, Inc.

life-saving or health-promoting interventions should not be denied for unfair reasons, including those with economic or social roots.

2. *Fostering Health Security.* One of the greatest threats to international health security arises from outbreaks of emerging and epidemic-prone diseases. Such outbreaks are occurring in increasing numbers, fueled by such factors as rapid urbanization, environmental mismanagement, the way food is produced and traded, and the way antibiotics are used and misused.

3. *Strengthening Health Systems.* Health services must reach poor and under-served populations. Health systems in many parts of the world are unable to do so. Areas being addressed include the provision of adequate numbers of appropriately trained staff, sufficient financing, suitable systems for collecting vital statistics, and access to appropriate technology including essential drugs.

4. *Harnessing Research, Information, and Evidence.* The WHO generates authoritative health information, in consultation with leading experts, to set norms and standards, articulate evidence-based policy options and monitor the evolving global heath situation.

5. *Enhancing Partnerships.* The WHO uses the strategic power of evidence to encourage partners implementing programs within countries to align their activities with best technical guidelines and practices, as well as with the priorities established by countries.

6. *Improving Performance.* The WHO participates in ongoing reforms aimed at improving its efficiency and effectiveness, both at the international level and within countries. The WHO aims to ensure that its strongest asset—its staff—works in an environment that is motivating and rewarding. The WHO plans its budget and activities through results-based management, with clear expected results to measure performance at country, regional, and international levels.

The WHO uses a process for quality assurance that includes the following principles:

- Implementing a reliance on the information supplied by the national drug regulatory authority.
- Fostering a general understanding of the quality control activities of the laboratory.
- Evaluating of information submitted by the laboratory.
- Assessing the consistency in quality control through compliance with good manufacturing practice(s) and WHO guidelines.

The International Organization for Standardization (ISO), which sets technical standards for a wide range of industries, developed the ISO 9000 standards relating to management systems to address objectives of satisfaction of customer's quality requirements, regulatory compliance, and meeting environmental goals.

Established in 1947, the ISO is a worldwide federation of national standards bodies from more than 148 countries. The mission of the ISO is to promote the development of standardization and related activities in the world with a view toward

(a) facilitating the international exchange of goods and services and (b) developing cooperation in the spheres of intellectual, scientific, technological, and economic activity. The ISO is a nongovernmental organization based in Geneva, Switzerland, and it is governed by a general assembly of its members. It undertakes the development of technical standards as its principal activity. By working through a network of international standardizing bodies, one from each member country, the work of the ISO produces international agreements that are published as International Standards and other types of ISO documents.

National standard bodies that wish to become members of the ISO must be national standards institutes or similar organizations, which are most representative of standardization in their country. In ISO terms, this works out as one member from each country, for a total of 148. Members can be full voting members, correspondent members (from countries that do not yet have fully developed national standards activity), or subscriber members (from countries with small economies that wish to maintain contact on issues of international standardization.)

It is representatives from these member bodies which collectively act to create standards. The standards are developed by technical committees comprising experts on loan from the industrial, technical, and business sectors. These individuals are often joined by substantive experts of the particular field that requires a new or amended standard set, to produce a well-rounded agreement. In this way, the ISO occupies a special position between the public and private sectors, thus acting as a bridging organization in which a consensus can be reached on solutions that meet both the requirements of business and the broader needs of society, such as the needs of stakeholder groups like consumers and users.

The ISO itself does not carry out certification of organizations complying with any set of ISO standards. Instead, certifications are carried out independently of the ISO by more than 750 certification bodies active around the world. These organizations are accredited by the member bodies of the ISO in each country in which they operate. In the United States, the American National Standards Institute (ANSI) is the sole US representative and dues-paying member of the ISO; and as a founding member of the ISO, ANSI plays an active role in its governance. ANSI is one of five permanent members to the governing ISO Council and is one of four permanent members of ISO's Technical Management Board. Through ANSI, the United States has immediate access to the ISO standards development processes. ANSI participates in 78% of all ISO technical committees and subcommittees, and ANSI holds the leadership roles for approximately 20% of all ISO technical committees and subcommittees.

At the outset, ISO standards were geared to the needs of the technical industry. However, demand for "international consensus on good management practice" led the ISO to develop standards concerning management systems. These generic management principles in 1987 were adapted into a set of standards known as ISO 9000, which address the following:

- Satisfaction of customer's quality requirements
- Regulatory compliance
- Meeting environmental objectives

The ISO 9000 standards are actually a group of standards and guidelines relating to management systems that are derived from the collective wisdom and knowledge of the international experts who participate in the ISO Technical Committee *ISO/TC 176, Quality Management and Quality Assurance*. These ISO 9000 quality standards are based on the following eight principles:

- Customer Focus
- Leadership
- Involvement of People
- Process Approach
- System Approach to Management
- Continual Improvement
- Factual Approach to Decision-Making
- Mutually Beneficial Supplier Relationships

For data on the numbers of certifications being granted, ISO performs an annual survey requesting certification data from a variety of sources, including national standards institutes, accreditation and certification bodies, and regional databases. The worldwide total of certificates was 500,125 in 2003.

ISO 9000 has been in existence since 1947 and has been the subject of several studies of its effectiveness. There has been some debate as to whether ISO 9000 certification can be said to improve organizational performance. To some organizations that have become certified, the process has clear value in improving their accountability to the public.

ISO certifications can now be found throughout the business, manufacturing, and service sectors. ISO 9000 addresses "process" rather than "product"; and the ISO 9000 standards provide a benchmark, or a best practice model, against which an organization's processes and management systems can be evaluated.

However, according to many, compliance with ISO 9000 can in fact undermine an organization's performance. It has been claimed that ISO 9000 predictably causes people to do things that, at best, suboptimize their organization's performance and, at worst, make it considerably worse. Examples of suboptimal outcomes include a contractual attitude toward customers and the development of an ethos of inspection within organizations. Worse yet, ISO 9000 standards are claimed to fit hand-in-glove with mass production or command and control thinking. Control of work through specifying and inspecting procedures is a variation on the theme of designing work in functional specialties, separating decision-making from doing the work and giving managers the job of making decisions on the basis of output or budgetary information. Quality standards, if applied at all, need to look at an organization as a moving target and intricate system rather than a static model.

The Organization for Economic Cooperation and Development (OECD) brings together the governments of countries committed to democracy and the market economy from around the world to

- Support sustainable economic growth
- Boost employment

- Raise living standards
- Maintain financial stability
- Assist other countries' economic development
- Contribute to growth in world trade

The OECD defines itself as a forum of countries committed to democracy and the market economy, providing a setting to compare policy experiences, seek answers to common problems, identify good practices, and coordinate domestic and international policies. Its mandate covers economic, environmental, and social issues. It acts by peer pressure to improve policy and implement "soft law"—that is, nonbinding instruments that can occasionally lead to binding treaties. In this work, the OECD cooperates with businesses, trade unions, and other representatives of civil society. Collaboration at the OECD regarding taxation, for example, has fostered the growth of a global web of bilateral tax treaties. The OECD provides a setting where governments compare policy experiences, seek answers to common problems, identify good practice, and coordinate domestic and international policies.

The OECD promotes policies designed to do the following:

- Achieve the highest sustainable economic growth and employment and a rising standard of living in member countries, while maintaining financial stability, and thus contribute to the development of the world economy.
- Contribute to sound economic expansion in Member as well as nonmember countries in the process of economic development.
- Contribute to the expansion of world trade on a multilateral, nondiscriminatory basis in accordance with international obligations.

The US Food and Drug Administration's International Conference on Harmonization (ICH), has issued guidance for efficacy, safety, quality, and joint safety/efficacy. The International Conference on Harmonization of Technical Requirements for Registration of Pharmaceuticals for Human Use (ICH) is a unique project that brings together the regulatory authorities of Europe, Japan, and the United States and experts from the pharmaceutical industry in the three regions to discuss scientific and technical aspects of product registration.

The purpose is to make recommendations on ways to achieve greater harmonization in the interpretation and application of technical guidelines and requirements for product registration in order to reduce or obviate the need to duplicate the testing carried out during the research and development of new medicines.

The objective of such harmonization is a more economical use of human, animal, and material resources, along with the elimination of unnecessary delay in the global development and availability of new medicines while maintaining (a) safeguards on quality, safety, and efficacy and (b) regulatory obligations to protect public health.

CHAPTER 15

FUTURE

15.1 PREDICTING THE FUTURE

The eight strategies for cost containment—requirements clarification, auditing, Quality by Design, outsourcing, electronic submissions, simultaneous FDA and EMEA submissions, control of visits, and use of a risk analysis—each can result in significant reduction of the investment required to assure compliance with regulatory requirements and guidelines. By lowering those expenses without negatively affecting product quality a more successful balance between access to medical devices, biologics and pharmaceuticals and the safety of those products can be achieved.

There is another strategy, significantly less certain and more problematically attainable, that could, if successful, add significantly to the success of the access/safety balance. Regulatory costs could be very effectively contained if only we could clearly and accurately predict the future of regulation.

Since ancient times there have been two basic approaches to foretelling the future (somewhat facetiously), categorized as (a) gazing into crystal ball and (b) reading the intestines of sacrificed animals. The latter is by far the more reliable, and it is utilized here.

Crystal balls and their ilk—tarot cards, astrological signs, and so on—rely on some sort of divine providence to reveal events that have yet to occur. While the method may be valid, depending on the whims of gods and the accuracy of the reader, it is certainly unscientific and likely to be unreliable.

Consider instead the reading of goat intestines. While it too may seem (and may be disguised as) communication with divine powers, there is an alternate interpretation. In a pastoral society, randomly selecting a few members of the herd and checking for intestinal parasites, tumors, and other early signs of disease may well predict the economic future of the tribe. These very real and scientifically observable early warning signs can be extrapolated to provide a reasonably accurate picture of coming events. This technique predicts the future by carefully examining the trends of the present, projecting those trends forward.

Cost-Contained Regulatory Compliance: For the Pharmaceutical, Biologics, and Medical Device Industries, First Edition. Sandy Weinberg.
© 2011 John Wiley & Sons, Inc. Published 2011 by John Wiley & Sons, Inc.

15.2   FOUR MAJOR TRENDS

There are four major trends emerging within the FDA that are likely to produce significant effects on the future of regulation—and regulatory cost containment—in the pharmaceutical, biologics, and medical device industries. Created by external forces and impacting on all aspects of the agency, these trends are increased operational transparency, new triage of investigational and review resources, increased international harmonization, and forced updating of regulatory guidelines.

The FDA has launch a "transparency initiative," recognizing the need to shed light on the processes and evaluations that traditionally have been held behind closed doors. While many of these procedures are described in public information, those descriptions may be rather obscurely archived and difficult to find and review. Other procedures are undocumented, more a result of tradition and established protocol rather than formal adoption. Finally, some decisions may be made without either established or informal procedures, apparently a result of capricious or arbitrary action.

Concern that the lack of transparency makes it impossible for a representative of a regulated industry or the general public to distinguish the arbitrary from the unwritten from the obscure, this initiative is in effect trying to apply the same standards imposed on the pharmaceutical, biologics, and medical device industries on the agency itself. For regulated industries, all procedures must be documented in carefully reviewed and approved Standard Operating Procedures (SOPs). The mantra has long been "If it isn't documented, there is no evidence that it happened." By applying the same principle to the FDA, internal procedures once poorly documented or undocumented should be available to public review (presumably under the Freedom of Information Act) as agency SOPs. And decisions not based upon those SOPs, or upon any clear procedure, would be reviewed, identified, and reconsidered.

While the transparency initiative is still in its early steps—focusing on developing strategies for disseminating information and increasing communication—it is clear that its impact is potentially significant. Perhaps most dramatically in the area of submissions reviews, pre-submission publication of the clear criteria utilized by a review panels could be a valuable tool in fine-tuning applications and potentially controlling submissions costs.

The investigation triage is a result of the intersection of three competing vectors. Over the past decade the US Congress has significantly increased the responsibility of the Food and Drug Administration, adding to its already complex mission the control of pharmaceutical advertising, the regulation of tobacco products and nutriceuticals, and other areas of concern. At the same time the number of pharmaceutical, device, and biologics facilities (all included under FDA inspection/ investigation responsibilities) has increased dramatically. Yet despite the increased drains on agency resources, budgetary constraints have held growth to minimal levels. The responsibilities and the number of facilities are rapidly outpacing capacity.

These pressures are already producing some fissures, and future changes are inevitable. Facilities scheduled for visitation every one to two years are now visited every three to five years. Increasingly, the agency is de facto accepting the findings of outside auditors, reviewing their reports in lieu of making more detailed FDA investigations. And increased triage, as the agency spends its time and budget on "putting out fires" rather than developing long-term prevention strategies, is inevitable.

The trend toward international harmonization has been oozing forward with the speed of molasses and the organizational drive of a herd of cats for decades. Progress is hampered by differences in regulatory mission, clinical testing philosophy, political trade barrier issues, and ethnocentrism. Some progress has been made in the medical device arena, likely to be reversed by pending major revisions in the FDA's policy on medical devices. Little of significance has been accomplished.

While the trend is not likely to accelerate in the near future, a critical mass has been realized, prompted by changes in the global pharmaceutical, biologics, and device industries. As financial pressures force international companies to conserve funds, they strongly encourage harmonization of regulation. And as more clinical research is conducted internationally, and more Active Pharmaceutical Ingredients (API) are produced outside of the United States and Europe, harmonization increasingly becomes imperative.

Regulatory guidelines are revised and expanded periodically, for a variety of reasons. Some are simply outdated, as with computer validation guidelines that are based upon the assumptions of a sequential, linear "waterfall" model, rendered largely obsolete by new programming technologies such as prototyping. In other cases, revisions are needed because of new technologies in the subjects of the regulation, such as new generations in medical devices and new categories of nuclear drugs with very short life spans. In still other circumstances, new guidelines are necessitated by legislative fiat (tobacco additives), business trends (pharmaceutical direct-to-public advertising), and public policy (orphan drugs).

When Ronald Reagan was President, he bragged about a reduction in the pages of regulation issued by the Federal Government; in reality, the reduction was only in the quantity of new regulations annually produced. New regulations were added under Reagan, and the total number and extent of guidelines grew; only the rate of new releases was reduced to a small extent. Under every administration for at least the last 50 years the quantity of new FDA regulatory guidelines has increased, and that trend is likely to continue.

A new acceleration of guidelines, standards, and requirements is now moving through the pipeline. In part this bulge is a result of slowed release under the Bush II administration, and in part it is a result of the scheduled reexamination of the core Good Manufacturing Practices regulations (ultimately requiring revision on Good Laboratory Practices, Good Tissue Practices, Good Clinical Practices, etc.). In part the new guidelines will result from the Transparency Initiative; in part from new emerging technologies; and in part from public and legislative concerns about emerging diseases, new vaccines, and new devices.

Finally, the slow crawl of harmonization with EMEA and other international guidelines will force some new and revised FDA regulations; while the totality of US and European regulations may decrease, the quantity of US regulation will grow in the process. All in all, the third major future trend—toward new guidelines and regulations—seems inevitable.

15.3 IMPACT OF FUTURE TRENDS

What will be the impact of these four future trends—greater FDA transparency, resources triage, international harmonization, and increased regulation—on the six cost-containment strategies?

The clear identification of requirements, and operationalization of those requirements to specific situations, should prove a cost-containment maximizing strategy under two of the future trends: greater FDA transparency and increased regulation. International harmonization and resource triage should have an important but lesser impact on the requirements strategy.

Improved transparency will lead to the release of more guidelines and criteria utilized in inspections, investigation, and reviews. These templates will provide the checklists needed to assure that situation-specific requirements interpretations conform to agency expectations and will provide some insurance that interpreted requirements will pass FDA scrutiny. The combination will encourage the requirements strategy: As the approach grows in commonality, it will accordingly grow in acceptance.

Similarly, increased regulation, including revisions of major regulatory standards like the cGMPs, will make the self-regulation approach of the requirements strategy more efficient and more effective. Clear regulations lead to clear situational definitions, which provide clear self-regulatory guides. As more and more applicable revised standards are produced, the utilization of those standards for internal control becomes an increasingly manageable, and increasingly popular, strategy.

To a lesser degree, internal harmonization will provide some clarification of common guidelines for global companies trying to establish standards conforming to the expectations of multiple regulatory agencies. And as FDA resources are pulled in more and more directions, the acceptability of self-regulation in accordance with specific regulatory definitions will increasingly become a de facto necessity. The FDA will gladly accept this strategy (among others) because it will help the agency to ration resources.

Under the predicted future trends, the requirements strategy should increase in potential value, increase in popularity, increase in agency acceptability, and prove a significant advantage in regulatory cost containment.

The strategic use of outside auditors will similarly benefit from the developing future trends. Because FDA transparency results in release of additional explanatory documents providing details of FDA evaluation criteria, audits will be able to apply those criteria to their own investigations, more closely aligning FDA and outsider observations.

FDA budgetary limitations will force the agency to increasingly operate on the ISO 9000 model, recommending, requiring, or encouraging annual independent audits of manufacturing sites, laboratories, systems, and clinical sites. The agency will, in turn, focus attention on the credential review of the auditors and on scrutiny of audit reports.

Harmonization will not dramatically affect the audit strategy, though it may reduce the costs somewhat as redundant audits are eliminated. The reality, though, is that most auditors have conducted their own harmonizations and have performed routine audit against both FDA and EMEA standards.

Finally, increased regulation will make a natural and proportionate increase in audits. As soon as the FDA releases a new standard or guideline, regulated organizations will need to know whether or not they conform and will also need to know how to correct any deviations. The independent audit will provide the answers and will serve an important a cost-containing role.

Since Quality by Design is evolving, it will continue to ride the cutting edge as FDA policies and procedures advance. The effect will be most obvious with the future triage of FDA activities due to funding limitations. QbD provides enhanced oversight at reduced cost, and those same cost savings will be felt by the FDA. A QbD monitoring report can provide FDA confidence in system control without the expense of a lengthy site visit.

The future may bring a more dramatic use of QbD. In the power industry a new business model has arisen: companies like GE Energy place QbD-like monitors throughout a power plant and (from a single global monitoring center located outside of Atlanta) can provide quality control for facilities in Iowa, China, India, Brazil, and anywhere else. A regulator could visit that monitoring station (live or electronically) and observe operations at any facility.

While there are important business confidentiality issues to be addressed, it is potentially possible that a similar model could be applied to the pharmaceutical, medical device, and biologics manufacturing industries. An independent centralized monitoring organization could coordinate QbD reporting, allowing the FDA greater oversight at considerably reduced cost. And, of course, the compliance costs will be contained for the regulated industries as well.

The effects on the QbD strategy of increased transparency, international harmonization of standards, and increased regulation are difficult to predict until the QBD concept is further solidified.

An increase in FDA transparency would not have a significant impact on the strategy of outsourcing or on its success as a cost-containment measure. Similarly, the FDA's continuing and growing shortage of resources would not affect outsourcing either positively or negatively. To the degree that harmonization of international requirements encouraged organizations to expand their markets and enter both US and European marketplaces simultaneously, there might be a slight increase in the need for outsourcing, particularly on a short-term basis as companies once restricted to a single market developed in-house expertise in other geographic regions.

An increase in regulation, on the other hand, would significantly enhance the value of an outsourcing strategy. Short-term response to new areas of regulation would require a potentially significant increase in headcount, presumably on a temporary basis. And the overnight need to build expertise in newly regulated fields would create a high outsource demand.

Consider, for example, the FDA's decision to require testing and validation of computer systems in the early 1990s. Organizations whose computer expertise was limited to designers, operators, and coders suddenly found themselves with a need for regulatory experts with technical computer skills. The gap was filled by the emergence of a number of computer regulatory companies offering outsourcing (and auditing) services to the pharmaceutical, biologics, and device industries. Weinberg Associates, for example, employed more than 100 full-time experts in computer validation and regulation and served as outsourced resources to a wide range of blood processing, monoclonal, large and small molecule, and medical device organizations.

In the same manner, any significant new FDA regulation or category of regulation will create an immediate need for outside consultants who can provide previously unneeded (and underdeveloped) technical skills and who can help regulated companies evolve those skills in house. The outsource personnel provide an important cost containment by meeting the need on a short term basis, and by bringing the expertise in house on a continuing basis.

Electronic submissions will be strongly encouraged and enhanced under all of the predicted future developments. As review criteria and processes become more transparent, the development of submissions applications tailored to those processes, and providing electronic links to key reviewer questions, will grow in value. These improved electronic submissions will widen the review speed and hence cost advantage over paper submissions.

Continuing and growing shortages of resources at the FDA will make the electronic submissions, and particularly the hyperlink capability, a resource that will rapidly gain FDA preference and attention. It is likely, in fact, that the growing budgetary pressures on FDA will soon force a requirement for electronic submissions, or a surcharge for paper submissions.

As international harmonization grows, the cost-containment strategy of electronic submissions, coupled with the dual submission strategy, will allow full advantage at significant cost containment. The ultimate dream, a common "universal submission" either processed simultaneously by all national agencies or reviewed by a single international agency—perhaps the World Health Organization—would save billions of dollars globally.

Increased regulation would have an indirect impact on electronic submissions: As organizations struggle to meet new regulatory initiatives, the time and resource conserving nature of electronic submissions will become increasingly valued. And as submission standards evolve—perhaps with expanded "Phase Five" (long-term studies) clinical data—electronic submissions will grow in value: The more involved the application, the more advantage to the electronic streamlined submission.

The growing value of the international dual submission cost-containment strategy would flow almost entirely from increase regulatory harmonization, but that advantage would be significant. As previously described, the "holy grail" of international regulation of pharmaceutical, biologics, and medical device products is the dream of a single global submission. This dual or multiple submission strategy either to a single reviewer or to simultaneous review of identical applications is a long way off, hampered by cultural differences, trade issues, and ethnocentrism. But it is no less realistic a dream than was the EMEA 30 years ago; and that centralized European review system, supplanting nationalistic agencies in the United Kingdom, France, Germany, and so on, is now a functioning relation. So too, increased harmonization of regulations will lead short term to greater cost containment with a dual submission strategy and will potentially lead long term to a single application possibility.

15.4   CONCLUSION

Predicting the future has always been a tricky business. Even using the rational approach of examining the impact of continuing trends on future events can be skewed by unexpected events, catastrophes, and unrecognized vectors. Despite these concerns, however, certain reasonable expectations seem so highly likely as to act like certainties. As the old joke goes, "The race goes not always to the swift, but it's a good idea to bet that way."

On the meta level, future planning should be predicated on the assumption that cost containment will be a continuing issue. No doubt economic growth will replace recession fears, and the boom–bust cycle will wax and wane. But in good times and bad, conserving funds and avoiding unnecessary regulation expenses makes good policy. The cost of pharmaceuticals, medical devices, and biologics will always be an access issue, and minimizing costs to maximize access is an appropriate approach.

More fundamentally, the four trends of greater FDA transparency, resources triage, international harmonization, and increased regulation seem like safe bets. Transparency is a political mainstay of the Obama administration, supported by Congressional mandate. The need for regulatory triage to cope with increasing responsibility and limited budget has been a characteristic of the FDA for the past 100+ years, and so relief is lurking just over the horizon.

International harmonization is a long, slow path: Progress is steady, but moves at a pace that perceives snails as speedsters. But, like glaciers, harmonization continues to move forward and is unlikely to fully halt or to reverse direction. For better or worse, international harmonization of regulations is continuing reality.

So, too, regulation tends to increase despite the best intentions of reformers and the best rhetoric of politicos. Several new regulatory expansions are just ahead, including a major revision of the cGMPs (and subsequent updates of GLPs, GCPs, etc.). And new technologies will drive new regulations to assure managerial and quality control.

In this evolving world, with continuing pressures to contain regulatory costs while maintaining product quality, the strategies of establishing clear regulatory definitions employing outside auditors, exploring and experimenting with Quality by Design, outsourcing where appropriate, utilizing electronic submissions, and overlapping international submissions will prove effective and valuable. With careful consideration of these strategies and appropriate implementation where appropriate, the pharmaceutical, biologics, and medical devices industries should be able to contain regulatory costs while assure the quality of drug, vaccines, devices, and related products.

BIBLIOGRAPHY

Clinical Research Articles, Journals, and Statements

von Eshenbach, Andrew C., MD. Statement to the Senate Agriculture, Rural Development, Food and Drug Administration, and Related Agencies Appropriations Sub-Committee, July 2007.

Clinical Research and Regulatory Affairs is a peered reviewed international journal. Available at http://informahealthcare.com/crr

JAMA, the Journal of the American Medical Association, a weekly peered-reviewed medical journal published by AMA. Available at http://jama.ama-assn.org/

Kamm, J. Can You Win the Space Race? *Pharmaceutical Manufacturing*, May 2007.

Konsky, David. Comparative Risk Projects: A Methodology for Cross-Project Analysis of Human Health Risk Rankings, Resources for the Future, August 1999.

Snee, R. D., P. Cini, J. Kamm, and C. Meyers. Quality by Design—Shortening the Path to Acceptance, *Pharma Processing*, February 2008.

Weinberg, Sandy. A Model of Quality by Design (QbD) Implementation in a Pharmaceutical Manufacturing Process, *ISPE Annual Conference*, October 2008.

Weinberg, Sandy. Cost-Effective Compliance, *Scientific Computer and Instrumentation*, March 2003.

Weinberg, Sandy. Early Warning: Attitude Adjustment at FDA, *American Biotechnology Laboratory*, July 2003.

Weinberg, Sandy. Pharmaceutical CGMPs for the 21st Century: A Risk Based Approach, *US FDA*, 21 August 2002.

Weinberg, Sandy. Process Analytical Technology for Chromatography, *Journal of Chromatographic Sciences*, Vol. 44, March 2006.

Weinberg, Sandy. System Validation, GAMP Harmonization and PAT, CFPA, Amsterdam, NE, December 2008.

Weinberg, Sandy. The FDA Vector: Part 11, Risk-Based Changes, *American Biotechnology Laboratory*, May 2003.

United States Food and Drug Administration, FDA. Risk-Based Method for prioritizing CGMP Inspections of Pharmaceutical Manufacturing Sites—A Pilot Risk Ranking Model, US FDA, September 2004.

Cost-Contained Regulatory Compliance: For the Pharmaceutical, Biologics, and Medical Device Industries, First Edition. Sandy Weinberg.
© 2011 John Wiley & Sons, Inc. Published 2011 by John Wiley & Sons, Inc.

Clinical Research Books

O'Mera, Alex. *Chasing Medical Miracles*, Walker Publishing, Reno, NV, 2009.

ICH Harmonized Tripartite Guideline: Pharmaceutical Development Q8, Current *Step 4* version, November 10, 2005, p. 11.

Nee, R. D., L. B. Hare and J. R. Trout. *Experiments in Industry—Design, Analysis and Interpretation of Results*, Quality Press, Birmingham, AL, 1985.

Weinberg, Sandy. *GALP Regulatory Handbook*, Weinberg, Spelton & Sax, Inc., Boothwin, PA, 1994.

Weinberg, Sandy. *Guidebook for Drug Regulatory Submissions*, John Wiley & Sons, Hoboken, NJ, 2009.

Weinberg, Sandy. *Good Laboratory Practice Regulations*, 4th edition (Drugs and the Pharmaceutical Sciences), Informa Healthcare USA, Inc., New York, 2007.

Weinberg, Sandy. Regulation of Computer Systems, in *Computer Applications in Pharmaceutical Research and Development*, 633–648, Ekins, Sean, ed., John Wiley & Sons, Hoboken, NJ, 2006.

Guidance, Compliance, and Regulatory Information

Code of Federal Regulations: http://www.gpoaccess.gov/cfr/

Drug Information Association: http://www.diahome.org/DIAHome/Home.aspx

European Commission: http://ec.europa.eu/index_en.htm

European Medicines Agency: http://www.ema.europa.eu/

International Organization for Standardization (ISO): http://www.iso.org/iso/home.html

National Institute of Child Health and Human Development International Health Regulations (IHR): http://www.nichd.nih.gov/health/clinicalresearch/regulations/

Organisation for Economic Co-Operation and Development (OECD): http://www.oecd.org/home/

Scrip Clinical Research: http://www.scripclinicalresearch.com/regulatory/

US Department of Health and Human Services

US Food and Drug Administration (US FDA)

Center for Biologics Evaluation and Research (CBER): http://www.fda.gov/biologicsbloodvaccines/default.htm

Center for Drug Evaluation and Research (CDER): http://www.fda.gov/drugs/default.htm

Guidance, Compliance, and Regulatory Information: http://www.fda.gov/drugs/guidancecomplianceregulatoryinformation/default.htm

Inspections, Compliance, Enforcement, and Criminal Investigations: http://www.fda.gov/ICECI/ComplianceManuals/ComplianceProgramManual/default.htm

International Conference on Harmonisation (ICH) Guidance Documents: http://www.fda.gov/regulatoryinformation/guidances/ucm122049.htm

Legislation: http://www.fda.gov/RegulatoryInformation/Legislation/default.htm

Running Clinical Trials: http://www.fda.gov/ScienceResearch/SpecialTopics/RunningClinicalTrials/default.htm

US Department of State Freedom of Information Act (FOIA): http://www.state.gov/m/a/ips/

World Health Organization: http://www.who.int/ihr/en/

World Medical Association: http://www.wma.net/en/20activities/10ethics/index.html

Support and Guidance for Companies

Center for Professional Advancement: http://www.cfpa.com/

ClinReg Research, Inc.: http://clinicaltrialresearch.com/

International Conference on Harmonization (ICH) of Technical Requirements for Registration of Pharmaceuticals for Human Use: http://www.ich.org/cache/compo/ 276-254-1.html

Chapter 12 Contacts

Australia: Therapeutics Goods Administration (TGA)

Email: info@tga.gov.au

Tel: 1800 020 653 (free call within Australia)

Tel: 02 6232 8444 (switchboard)

Tel: 02 6232 8610 (for publications enquiries)

Fax: 02 6203 1605

Post: TGA, PO Box 100, Woden ACT 2606, Australia

Brazil: Sanitary Surveillance Agency (Anvisa)

Email: infovisa@anvisa.gov.br.

Ombudsman's Office through phone number (61) 448-1235, 448-1464 or through phone/fax 448-1144

China: State Food and Drug Agency (SFDA)

State Food and Drug Administration

A38, Beilishi Road

Beijing 100810, People's Republic of China

Fax: 86-010-68310909

Email: inquires@sda.gov.cn

European Union: European Medicines Agency (EMEA)

European Medicines Agency

7 Westferry Circus

Canary Wharf

London E14 4HB

United Kingdom

Telephone switchboard: +44 (0)20 7418 8400

Web site: www.ema.europa.eu

France: Agence Française de Sécurité Santaire des Produits de Santé (AFSSAPS)

143-147, Blvd Anatole France

93285 Saint-Denis Cedex France

www.afssaps.fr

Tel: +33 155 87 3000

Fax: +33 155 87 3172

Germany: Federal Institute for Drugs and Medical Devices (Bundesinstitut für Arzneimittel und Medizinprodukte, BfArM)

Bundesinstitut für Arzneimittel und Medizinprodukte

Kurt-Georg-Kiesinger-Allee 3

D-53175 Bonn, Germany

Tel: +49 (0)228 99-307-0

Telefax: +49 (0)228 99-307-5207

E-mail: poststelle@bfarm.de

India: Central Drug Standard Control Organisation (CDSCO)

Central Drugs Standard Control Organisation

Directorate General of Health Services

Ministry of Health and Family Welfare

Government of India

FDA Bhavan, ITO, Kotla Road

New Delhi 110002, India

Phone: 91-11-2323695 / 23236975

Fax: 91-11-23236973

Israel: Description of Ministry of Health (IMOH)

Ministry of Health

2 Ben Tabai St.

Jerusalem, Israel 91010

Tel: 972-2-6705705

Tel: 972-2-5681200

Email: pniot@moh.health.gov.il

Japan: Description of Pharmaceuticals and Medical Devices Agency (PMDA)

Pharmaceuticals and Medical Devices Agency

Shin-Kasumigaseki Building

3-3-2 Kasumigaseki

Chiyoda-ku, Tokyo 100-0013,Japan

Tel: +81-3-3506-9456

Fax: +81-3-3506-9572

E-mail: info.pmda.f10@pmda.go.jp

Korea (South): Description of Korea Food and Drug Administration (KDFA)

194 Tongiro

Eunpyeoung-gu

Seoul 122-704, Republic of Korea

Email: kdfa@kdfa@go.kr

Switzerland: Description of Swissmedic

Swiss Agency for Therapeutic Products

Hallerstrasse 7

CH-3000 Bern 9, Switzerland

Phone: +41 31 322 02 11

Fax: +41 31 322 02 12

United Kingdom: Description of Medicines and Healthcare Products Regulatory Agency (MHRA)

10-2 Market Towers

1 Nine Elms Lane

London SW8 5NQ, United Kingdom

Tel: 020 7084 2000 (weekdays 0900–1700)

Tel: 020 7210 3000 (other times)

Fax: 020 7084 2353

Email: info@mhra.gsi.gov.uk

INDEX

Information in tables is denoted by *t*.

Cost-Contained Regulatory Compliance: For the Pharmaceutical, Biologics, and Medical Device Industries, First Edition. Sandy Weinberg.
© 2011 John Wiley & Sons, Inc. Published 2011 by John Wiley & Sons, Inc.

Printed in the United States
By Bookmasters